LIVING THERAPY SERIES

Counselling for Progressive Disability

Person-Centred Dialogues

Richard Bryant-Jefferies

Radcliffe Medical Press
Oxford ● San Francisco

Radcliffe Medical Press Ltd
18 Marcham Road
Abingdon
Oxon OX14 1AA
United Kingdom

www.radcliffe-oxford.com
The Radcliffe Medical Press electronic catalogue and online ordering facility.
Direct sales to anywhere in the world.

British Library Cataloguing in Publication Data

A catalogue record for this book is available from the British Library.

ISBN 1 85775 898 6

Typeset by Aarontype Limited, Easton, Bristol
Printed and bound by TJ International Ltd, Padstow, Cornwall

Contents

Foreword

Wow! This was my first reaction and it came before I actually reached the text! In the preface and introduction to this book, which is one of a series of books written by author Richard Bryant-Jefferies, I'd found a description of what the book set out to do. Not normally one to read such sections of a book, preferring to get to the substance of a book within which to dip, I was astounded and not a little awed at what was to be achieved.

Having trained in humanistic psychology, I currently identify my practice as based on the person-centred principles of acceptance, respect and empathy, with additional intervention that I feel are in harmony both with each other and this base philosophy. To discover that Richard was to demonstrate a purely person-centred approach to something as complex as disability – progressive disability – was quite intriguing.

Both the clients are fictional, Richard tells us, and yet as I read, I had a strong sense of the reality of the clients' stories. As a busy professional and an equally busy person, I am aware that I am also working through my own disability, struggling at times to reconcile my perception of myself as an active, healthy person with the newer understanding that I face a daily struggle against pain and disability, and cannot behave as before. Rather than dipping into the text, as I so often do with much of my counselling library (yes, I am a book addict and cannot resist buying both counselling and supervision books as well as novels), I found myself reading this one as if it really was a novel, keen to share the experience in the therapeutic encounter.

The book sets out to share two things: a journey of deepening understanding regarding the progression of a disabling illness through the words of the two clients; and the power of the purely person-centred approach to create therapeutic movement. Additionally, there are reflective insertions that share the process of this counselling, and give the reader a real sense of how person-centredness, by simply 'being', is able to support movement by the client.

By including supervision sessions that mirror the counselling technique and allow the counsellor to explore his responses to the client work. Richard gives a very real sense of the empowering qualities of person-centred counselling. A good read for anyone in the helping and caring professions, and particularly for students learning to be counsellors, the book demonstrates very clearly how the reflective responses of the counsellor enable the clients to see their own process and by working with this they achieve a greater understanding and acceptance of themselves.

I am particularly impressed with the way the dialogue, through each chapter, demonstrates a purity of person-centred technique and a feeling of how enabling this process seems to be for client, counsellor and supervisor. However, my own experience of counselling work in all its forms has taught me that many clients struggle with the need to work through their difficulties, and that this of itself is almost as disabling as the problem situation itself.

In Richard's rich narrative thread, there is for me a thrill at seeing the client (Pauline) acknowledging this, and it being reflected back, '*But it leaves you feeling more able to face things.*' I shall continue to hear that sentence, as a wonderful encapsulation of the purpose of my own counselling and supervisory work ... that my purpose is not to cure, but to enable.

But, I write those words as a professional counsellor and one-time lecturer. I am very aware of the jargon words I've used, and that you hear little of the real me responding to what I read. So, to really tell it how it is, I think you need to know that if you choose this book, you won't merely dip into it for quotes or methodology. You will be, as I was, caught up in the story, wanting to know what happens next and finding yourself reluctant to put the book down.

As they say in other areas of recommendation, this book is a cracking read. You *will* be caught up in its depth and power, and you will come to a real appreciation of how much someone can achieve, even with a life-changing disability, simply by being actively listened to!

Justine Oldfield-Rowell
January 2004

Justine Oldfield-Rowell is a BACP Registered Therapist and BAPC Registered Supervisor. She has lectured in counselling in an FE College but now works full-time in independent practice. She is Chair of the Personal, Relationship and Group-work Division of the British Association for Counselling and Psychotherapy.

Foreword

When a disability is or becomes part of a person's life, this often implies a strong experience of loneliness and isolation for many people. Not to be like others means not to be part of a community. And the anxiety which a disability, whether progressive or congenital, raises in other people often leads them to turn away, avoiding the awareness that this might happen to anyone. The lack of contact and empathy makes it harder for the person to cope with the hardship this disability can lead to.

When there is such a drastic change in a person's life, this affects his or her self-image and self-esteem, and it requires entirely new ways of coping with life. It means a loss of security and a certainty in life which until then was experienced as natural and was not really questioned. It also leads to a huge anxiety, even more so as the physical process is one of progressive deterioration. Acceptance and empathy can help the person to process these feelings which come with the illness and disability, and to integrate the changes.

Since 1991 I have worked with children, adolescents and adults with different kinds of disability in a variety of therapeutic settings (as well as working as a supervisor of professional carers of people with disabilities and counselling parents of disabled adults). From my own experience I can well appreciate the contribution that the person-centred psychotherapist can make in supporting and enabling people affected by disability to gradually develop a new way of being.

The literature about person-centred theory is very rich. The section of publications which focus on practical person-centred work is certainly enriched by this volume. Maybe the avoidance of this subject in life is one of the reasons why there is not much theoretical reflection about working with people with disabilities. This book brings the issue closer to us, showing that the person with the disability is not so different in his or her way of experiencing and reflecting from others. The author, who was personally affected by his father's progressive disability, writes in such a way that any reader reaches an understanding of what is going on in each client, and also between the client and the therapist. It is almost as if we are present in the session and can read the minds of both therapist and client. Even though the clients go through difficult processes, the way we can follow them in their emotional development may take away the anxiety the issue of a progressive disability raises in each of us, as gradually we come closer to this person in the course of the process.

The author has successfully undertaken the difficult task of trying to bring the practice of person-centred psychotherapy closer to the reader. He has done this in such a way that it is possible to follow the process of the client step by step. The book presents two counselling processes which unfold throughout the chapters. In between, the author has inserted small frames in which he zooms in on what is happening in the counselling relationship. At times he refers to person-centred theory or adds explanations with clinical content. The counselling process is reflected upon in supervision sessions which give a good insight into person-centred supervision. Thus, the reader can learn about three aspects at the same time: the process a progressive disability induces, a person-centred way of working with that issue and person-centred supervision.

While the book will be useful to any person-centred psychotherapist working with clients who are struggling with such life issues as demonstrated here, it will be invaluable to newcomers to the person-centred approach and to trainees who are developing their practical skills for person-centred work. I am convinced that this book will not only make the person-centred approach accessible to a wider audience, but also increase the general acceptance and empathy for persons with disabilities.

Elisabeth Zinschitz
President of OEGWG (Austrian Client-Centred Association)
Clinical Director of Child Protection Centre, Vienna
Client-centred therapist in private practice
January 2004

Preface

While I have not myself experienced multiple sclerosis (MS), I have lived in a family affected by progressively disability. My father fought a 40-year battle against progressive disability from arthritis. I have allowed this experience to inform me but have sought not to draw directly from this. I have also counselled people with arthritic conditions, and have learned to appreciate the personal nature of pain, the struggle to come to terms with a progressively disabling disease, the stressful impact it can have on family and close friends, and the positive and creative ways that people have responded.

This book sets out to provide the reader with an experience of working with a person suffering progressive disability, both in the early stages and at an advanced and more disabling stage, from a person-centred theoretical perspective. It aims to enable the reader to enter into the world of the person who is being confronted with pain and loss of mobility, fear for the future, anger at what has happened and is happening, sadness for lost dreams and hopes. It also offers the opportunity to experience the thoughts, feelings and reactions of the counsellor who is working with them. It does not seek to be simply a book about counselling people suffering from MS. Feelings and experiences such as pain, loss, fear, anger, rage, depression, anxiety and hopelessness, among others, are factors that can emerge from being confronted with the reality of any progressive disability.

Included is material to inform the training process of counsellors and many others who seek to work with people experiencing pain and/or progressive disability. *Counselling for Progressive Disability: person-centred dialogues* is intended as much for experienced counsellors as it is for trainees. It provides real insight into what can occur during counselling sessions, based on work with two clients at different stages in their life: the experience of symptoms indicative of a progressive disabling condition; and at a time when the dilemma as to whether to accept the need to use a wheelchair is faced. Reflections on the process and points for discussion are included to stimulate further thought and debate.

Counselling for Progressive Disability: person-centred dialogues will also be of value to the many healthcare and social care professionals who work with people with progressive disability. For all these professionals, the text demystifies what can occur in therapy, and at the same time provides useful ways of working that may be used by professionals other than counsellors.

I hope, as well, that this book will find its way not only into neurology depart-ments, and indeed all medical specialities where progressive disability is an issue, but also into rehabilitation and occupational therapy units.

Richard Bryant-Jefferies
January 2004

About the author

Richard Bryant-Jefferies qualified as a person-centred counsellor/therapist in 1994 and remains passionate about the application and effectiveness of this approach. His first experience of counselling was as a volunteer and home visitor for an arthritis support group. He chose this area of work mainly because his own home experience had been one largely affected by his father's struggle with ankylosing spondylitis, osteoarthritis and rheumatoid arthritis.

Between early 1995 and mid-2003 Richard worked at a community drug and alcohol service in Surrey, and more recently he has taken up a position managing substance misuse services in a London borough. He has experience of both counselling and supervision.

Richard had his first book on a counselling theme published in 2001, *Counselling the Person Beyond the Alcohol Problem* (Jessica Kingsley Publishers), providing theoretical yet practical insights into the application of the person-centred approach within the context of the 'cycle of change' model that has been widely adopted to describe the process of change in the field of addiction. Since then he has been writing for the *Living Therapy* series (Radcliffe Medical Press), producing an ongoing series of person-centred dialogues: *Problem Drinking, Time Limited Therapy in Primary Care, Counselling a Survivor of Child Sexual Abuse, Counselling a Recovering Drug User* and *Counselling Young People*. The aim of the series is to bring the reader a direct experience of the counselling process, an exposure to the thoughts and feelings of both client and counsellor as they encounter each other on the therapeutic journey, and an insight into the value and importance of supervision.

Richard is keen to bring the experience of the therapeutic process, from the standpoint and application of the person-centred approach, to a wider audience. He is convinced that the principles and attitudinal values of this approach and the emphasis it places on the therapeutic relationship are key to helping people create greater authenticity both in themselves and in their lives, leading to a fuller and more satisfying human experience.

Acknowledgements

In writing this book I would like to express my gratitude to Caron Oyston, who as well as being a counsellor, supervisor and trainer also has MS; and Elen Sentier, who was a counsellor for a number of years and is now an author, and suffers with arthritis. Both contributed helpful and insightful feedback on the draft for this book. Thank you both.

I would also like to thank, once again, the series editor, Maggie Pettifer, for her continued support, energy, enthusiasm and encouragement in the writing of the *Living Therapy* series.

Last, but certainly not least, I want to thank the many people that I have met over the years who have been faced with the challenge of a progressive disability – in particular my father, Philip, to whom I dedicate this book. Whilst part of me is sad he is not alive to read it, another part of me knows that if he had been alive today it would have meant a few more years of pain and struggle. I would not wish that on him, or on anyone.

Introduction

In many ways this book is perhaps unique insofar as it is written to offer the reader an opportunity to experience and to appreciate, through dialogue, some of the diverse and challenging issues that can arise when working with a person who is confronted with the reality of progressive disability. It is composed of fictitious dialogues between fictitious clients and their counsellors, and between the counsellors and their supervisors. Within the dialogues are woven the reflective thoughts and feelings of the client, the counsellor and the supervisor, along with boxed comments on the process and references to person-centred theory.

The book has been written with the aim of demonstrating the counsellor's application of the person-centred approach (PCA) – a theoretical approach to counselling that has, at its heart, the power of the therapeutic relationship, offering the client an experience through which greater potential for authentic living may emerge – when working with people who have a disabling health condition. The approach is widely used by counsellors working in the UK today: in a membership survey in 2001 by the British Association for Counselling and Psychotherapy, 35.6 per cent of those responding claimed to work to the person-centred approach, while 25.4 per cent identified themselves as psychodynamic practitioners.

The reader may find it takes a while to adjust to the dialogue format. Many of the responses offered by the two counsellors, Maureen and Jim, are reflections of what their respective clients, Gerry and Pauline, have said. This is not to be read as conveying a simple repetition of the client's words. Rather, the counsellor seeks to voice empathic responses, often with a sense of 'checking out' that they are hearing accurately what the client is saying. The client says something; the counsellor then conveys that they have heard it, sometimes with the same words, sometimes including a sense of what they feel may be being communicated through the client's tone of voice, facial expression or simply the atmosphere of the moment. The client is then enabled to confirm that they have been heard accurately, or correct the counsellor in their perception. The client may then explore more deeply what they have been saying or move on, in either case with a sense that they have been heard and warmly accepted. To draw this to the reader's attention, I have attempted to highlight some of the reflections that occur throughout the work by inserting Maureen's and Jim's reflective thoughts in boxes throughout the dialogue.

The supervision sessions are included to offer the reader insight into the nature of therapeutic supervision in the context of the counselling profession, a method of supervising that I term 'collaborative review'. For many trainee counsellors, the use of supervision can be something of a mystery, and it is hoped that this book will go a long way to unravelling this. In the supervision sessions I seek to demonstrate the application of the supervisory relationship. My intention is to show how supervision of the counsellor is very much a part of the process of enabling a client to work through issues that, in this case, relate to pain and progressive disability.

Many professions do not recognise the need for some form of personal and process supervision, and often what is offered is line management. However, counsellors are required to receive regular supervision in order to explore the dynamics of the relationship with the client, the impact of the work on the counsellor and on the client, to receive support, and to provide an opportunity for an experienced co-professional to monitor the supervisee's work in relation to ethical standards and codes of practice. The supervision sessions are included because they are an integral part of the therapeutic process. It is also hoped that they will help readers from other professions to recognise the value of some form of supportive and collaborative supervision in order to help them become more authentically present with their own clients.

Merry (2002) describes what he terms 'collaborative inquiry' as a 'form of research or inquiry in which two people (the supervisor and the counsellor) collaborate or co-operate in an effort to understand what is going on within the counselling relationship and within the counsellor'. There are, of course, as many models of supervision as there are models of counselling. In this book the supervisor is seeking to apply the attitudinal qualities of the person-centred approach.

It is the norm for all professionals working in the healthcare and social care environment in this age of regulation to be formally accredited or registered and to work to their own professional organisation's code of ethics or practice. For instance, registered counselling practitioners with the British Association for Counselling and Psychotherapy are required to have regular supervision and continuing professional development to maintain registration. While professions other than counsellors will gain much from this book in their work with patients or clients with progressive disability, it is essential that they follow the standards, safeguards and ethical codes of their own professional organisation, and are appropriately trained and supervised to work with their clients.

All characters in this book are fictitious and are not intended to bear resemblance to any particular person or persons.

The person-centred approach

The person-centred approach (PCA) was formulated by Carl Rogers, and references are made to his ideas within the text of the book. However, it will be helpful for readers who are unfamiliar with this way of working to have an appreciation of its theoretical base.

Rogers proposed that certain conditions, when present within a therapeutic relationship, would enable the client to develop towards what he termed 'fuller functionality'. Over a number of years he refined these ideas, which he defined as 'the necessary and sufficient conditions for constructive personality change'. These he described as follows.

1 Two persons are in psychological contact.
2 The first, whom we shall term the client, is in a state of incongruence, being vulnerable or anxious.
3 The second person, whom we shall term the therapist, is congruent or integrated in the relationship.
4 The therapist experiences unconditional positive regard for the client.
5 The therapist experiences an empathic understanding of the client's internal frame of reference and endeavours to communicate this experience to the client.
6 The communication to the client of the therapist's empathic understanding and unconditional positive regard is to a minimal degree achieved. (Rogers, 1957, p. 96)

The first necessary and sufficient condition given for constructive personality change is that of 'two persons being in psychological contact'. However, although he later published this as simply 'contact' (Rogers, 1959), it is suggested (Wyatt and Sanders, 2002, p. 6) that this was actually written in 1953–54. They quote Rogers as defining contact in the following terms: 'Two persons are in psychological contact, or have the minimum essential relationship when each makes a perceived or subceived difference in the experiential field of the other' (Rogers, 1959, p. 207). A recent exploration of the nature of psychological contact from a person-centred perspective is given by Warner (2002).

Rogers defined empathy as 'entering the private perceptual world of the other ... being sensitive, moment by moment, to the changing felt meanings which flow in this other person ... It means sensing meanings of which he or she is scarcely aware, but not trying to uncover totally unconscious feelings' (Rogers, 1980, p. 142) It is a very delicate process, and it provides, I believe, a foundation block. The counsellor's role is primarily to establish empathic rapport and communicate empathic understanding to the client.

Within this relationship the counsellor seeks to maintain an attitude of unconditional positive regard towards the client and all that they disclose. This is not 'agreeing with'; it is simply warm acceptance. Rogers wrote, 'when the therapist is experiencing a positive, acceptant attitude towards whatever the client *is* at that moment, therapeutic movement or change is more likely to occur' (Rogers, 1980, p. 116). Mearns and Thorne suggest that 'unconditional positive regard is the label given to the fundamental attitude of the person-centred counsellor towards her client. The counsellor who holds this attitude deeply values the humanity of her client and is not deflected in that valuing by any particular client behaviours. The attitude manifests itself in the counsellor's consistent acceptance of and enduring warmth towards her client' (Mearns and Thorne, 1988, p. 59).

Last, but by no means least, is the state of being that Rogers referred to as congruence, but which has also been described in terms of 'realness', 'transparency', 'genuineness' and 'authenticity'. Indeed, Rogers wrote that '... genuineness, realness or congruence ... this means that the therapist is openly being the feelings and attitudes that are flowing within at the moment ... the term transparent catches the flavour of this condition'. Putting this into the therapeutic setting, we can say that 'congruence is the state of being of the counsellor when her outward responses to her client consistently match the inner feelings and sensations which she has in relation to her client' (Mearns and Thorne, 1999, p. 84).

I would suggest that any congruent expression by the counsellor of their feelings or reactions has to emerge through the process of being in therapeutic relationship with the client. It is a disciplined response and not an open door to endless self-disclosure. Congruent expression is perhaps most appropriate and therapeutically valuable where it is informed by the existence of an empathic understanding of the client's inner world, and is offered in a climate of a genuine warm acceptance towards the client.

PCA regards the relationship that we have with our clients and the attitude that we hold within that relationship to be key factors. In my experience, many adult psychological difficulties develop out of life experiences that involve problematic, conditional or abusive relational experiences. This can be centred in childhood or later in life. What is important is that the individual is left, through relationships that have a negative conditioning effect, with a distorted perception of themselves and their potential as a person. I see many people who have learned from childhood experience beliefs such as 'I can never be good enough to be praised for what I have achieved; I never match my parents' expectations' or 'No one was ever there for me when I was hurting; perhaps I am unlovable'. The result is a loss of a positive sense of self, and the individual adapts to maintain the newly learned concept of self. This is then lived out, possibly throughout life, with the person seeking to satisfy what they have come to believe about themselves: being unable to achieve, feeling unable or undeserving to be loved, though perhaps in both cases maintaining a constant desperation to receive what they never had. Yet, perversely, they may then sabotage any possibility of gaining what they want in order to maintain the negatively conditioned sense of self and the sense of satisfaction that this gives them because they have developed such a strong identity with it.

It is my belief that by offering someone a non-judgemental, warm, accepting and authentic relationship, the person can grow into a fresh sense of self in which their potential as a person can become more fulfilled. Such an experience fosters an opportunity for the client to redefine themselves as they experience the presence of the therapist's congruence, empathy and unconditional positive regard. This process can take time. Often the personality change that is required to sustain a shift away from what have been termed 'conditions of worth' requires a lengthy period of therapeutic work, bearing in mind that the person may be struggling to unravel a sense of self that has been developed, sustained and reinforced for many decades of life.

The term 'conditions of worth' applies to the conditioning that is frequently present in childhood, and at other times in life, when a person experiences that their worth is conditional on their doing something, or behaving, in a certain way. This is usually to satisfy someone else's needs, and can be contrary to the client's own sense of what would be a satisfying experience. The values of others become a feature of the individual's structure of self. The person moves away from being true to themselves, learning instead to remain 'true' to their conditioned sense of worth. This state of being in the client is challenged by the person-centred therapist by offering them unconditional positive regard and warm acceptance. Such a therapist, by genuinely offering these therapeutic attitudes, provides the client with an opportunity to be exposed to what may be a new experience or one that in the past they have dismissed, preferring to stay with that which matches and therefore reinforces their conditioned sense of worth and sense of self. Unconditional positive regard and warm acceptance offered consistently over time can, and does, enable clients to begin to question their beliefs about themselves and to begin to build into their structure of self the capacity to see and experience themselves as being of value for who they are. It enables them to liberate themselves from the constraints of patterns of conditioning.

A crucial feature or factor in this process is the presence of what Rogers termed 'the actualizing tendency', a tendency towards fuller and more complete person-hood with an associated greater fulfilment of their potentialities. The role of the person-centred counsellor is to provide the facilitative climate within which this tendency can work constructively. 'The therapist trusts the actualizing tendency of the client and truly believes that the client who experiences the freedom of a fostering psychological climate will resolve his or her own problems' (Bozarth, 1998, p. 4). This is fundamental to the application of the person-centred approach. Rogers (1986, p. 198) wrote: 'the person-centred approach is built on a basic trust in the person ... (It) depends on the actualizing tendency present in every living organism – the tendency to grow, to develop, to realize its full potential. This way of being trusts the constructive directional flow of the human being towards a more complex and complete development. It is this directional flow that we aim to release.'

The therapeutic relationship is central. A therapeutic approach such as person-centred affirms that it is not what you do so much as 'how you are' with your client that is therapeutically significant, and this 'how you are' has to be received by the client. Gaylin (2001, p. 103) highlights the importance of client perception. 'If clients believe that their therapist is working on their behalf – if they perceive caring and understanding – then therapy is likely to be successful. It is the condition of attachment and the perception of connection that have the power to release the faltered actualization of the self.' He goes on to stress how 'we all need to feel connected, prized – loved', describing human beings as 'a species born into mutual interdependence', and that there 'can be no self outside the context of others'. He highlights that 'loneliness is dehumanizing and isolation anathema to the human condition. The relationship,' he suggests, 'is what psychotherapy is all about.'

There is currently growing interest in, and much debate about, theoretical developments within the person-centred world and its application. Discussions on the theme of Rogers' therapeutic conditions presented by various key members of the person-centred community have recently been published (Bozarth and Wilkins, 2001; Haugh and Merry, 2001; Wyatt, 2001; Wyatt and Sanders, 2002). Mearns and Thorne (2000) have recently produced a timely publication revising and developing key aspects of person-centred theory. Wilkins (2003) has produced a book that addresses most effectively many of the criticisms levelled against person-centred working. It seems to me that the relational component of the person-centred approach, based on the presence of the core conditions, is emerging strongly as a counter to the sense of isolation that frequently accompanies deep psychological and emotional problems, and the increase in what I would term a 'rabid inauthenticity' within materialistic societies as we enter the 21st century.

This is obviously a very brief introduction to the approach. Person-centred theory continues to develop as practitioners and theoreticians consider its application in various fields of therapeutic work and extend our theoretical understanding of developmental and therapeutic processes. At times it feels like it has become more than just individuals; rather it feels like a group of colleagues, based around the world, working together to penetrate deeper towards a more complete theory of the human condition. It is an exciting time.

Pain and disability

The person faced with the prospect of progressive disability is likely to pass through a range of reactions: 'Why me?', 'How will I cope with the pain?', 'I'm going to lose so much', 'I want to hide away', 'Will my marriage survive it?', 'What about sex?', 'I'll lose my job', 'I don't want to be labelled "disabled"'. There will be many more, each set of reactions unique to the person who has been given a disabling diagnosis.

What the effects will be, only time can tell. But what is sure is that the person will be confronted with the need for adaptation, with a need to make sometimes small, sometimes far-reaching adjustments in their life. Progressive disability is like a conveyor belt of change, of struggling to cling to independence, and reaching critical points when the onward march of the condition requires an acceptance that some of the things that were part of the person's life are now out of reach.

Losses can be wide-ranging and, in a very real sense, need to be grieved over individually (Segal, 2002). It may be the loss of what was – pain-free mobility, an identity rooted in a self-concept of being healthy. It could well undermine self-confidence and self-esteem. It could be a loss of dreams and hopes for the future: plans for a lifestyle that is now out of reach, or simply any plans, because suddenly there is a struggle to imagine what the future might be like. Or the future might look all too clear, a limited lifestyle and probable reliance on a wheelchair to get around. Previous unresolved losses that may have little or nothing to do with the disabling condition may come sharply to the fore as well, needing to be acknowledged and processed.

The uncertainty of life is suddenly exacerbated. What will happen? How will it be? Needing to know conflicts with not wanting to know. What choices do I make? What is for the best? Some people will react by not wanting to know, going into denial and staying there for some time; others move into a frantic phase of information gathering, wanting to know exactly what they are up against. And, of course, there are many points along the continuum between these two.

Is disability much more recognised and accepted in our society? It is one thing to have ramps for access, dipping buses and disabled toilets. Yes, they are important. But at least as important, and probably more so, are the human reactions from other people, the expressions on people's faces in the street, the reactions of work colleagues who may not believe you are in pain because there is no visible wound.

Working with a group of people for whom there is a high likelihood that things can only get worse is a challenge. The person-centred counsellor will seek to understand the person as they are experiencing themselves, with all the fears, anxieties, losses and uncertainties that progressive disability can bring. The counsellor must expect to be affected by entering this inner, private world of their client. The client can be feeling overwhelmed, and so can the counsellor.

While counselling can be at risk of becoming diagnosis- or symptom-centred, the person-centred counsellor seeks to see the client as not so much 'a disabled person' as 'a person with a disability'. Their focus and emphasis lies on the personhood of the individual with whom they are building the therapeutic relationship, the disabling condition being one factor – and in this context a major factor – influencing and shaping their client's sense of self.

PART I

Coming to terms with the diagnosis of progressive disability

CHAPTER 1

Setting the scene

Gerry had lived a fairly normal life really; he was now in his early thirties and had established himself in a large organisation in a fairly senior management position. He had worked for the same company since leaving school and had worked his way up. He felt good about his work, enjoyed the people that he worked with and felt secure in his position.

He lived with his wife, Carol, and their two children on the edge of town. They owned a detached house and Gerry enjoyed maintaining their garden, which he had landscaped himself since they had moved there two years ago.

His children were both still at school. Amy was ten and Darius was eight. Everything seemed so secure and certain – that was until he started getting discomfort in his lower back and legs, and headaches. It hadn't begun as a problem; in fact, he'd had twinges on and off for years, but had put it down to overdoing it a bit, or the weather. And maybe that was still true. But it had become worse and at one point he had found himself struggling to walk. His legs just didn't seem to respond or, at least, not as he was used to. Just didn't seem to have the same mobility. It had really scared him and had taken him by surprise. He had gone to the doctor who had referred him to the neurologist. He was waiting to hear when his appointment would be. Meanwhile, because Gerry seemed to be really struggling emotionally with his symptoms, the GP had also referred him to the counsellor for some emotional support.

Counselling session 1: the client struggles to make visible his fear

It had been a two-week wait to see the counsellor. Gerry's symptoms had got worse, though not consistently so. The constant pain in his head, behind his eyes, was getting him down, and the shooting pains in his legs were affecting his movement. The GP had suggested he see a counsellor for a few sessions. Gerry was now sitting in the waiting room at the health centre waiting to be seen.

He heard his name being called and he turned around to see who had called him.
A woman in her fifties, thought Gerry, was smiling his way. 'Hi, Gerry?'
'Yes.'
'Hi, would you like to come this way?' Maureen didn't mention she was the counsellor, wanting to maintain confidentiality. There were other people in the
waiting room and not everyone wanted it to be known that they were attending counselling.

Maureen began by explaining about confidentiality and describing the nature
and purpose of counselling, ensuring that Gerry was informed and therefore
able to give informed consent to 'treatment'. Maureen never thought of herself
as offering 'treatment' – it just did not fit with her philosophy as a person-
centred counsellor – but she was aware that clients had a right to know what
they were agreeing to.

Gerry himself wasn't too interested. He just knew he wanted someone to talk to.
He knew he was struggling, could see a very bleak future and his mood had slid
down a great deal over the past couple of weeks to the point that he was really
doing very little at home and was just not taking interest in very much at all.
He was really struggling to move around, and kept getting stabbing pains running down his spine and his legs. He often looked down at his legs and wondered
if they were really his. They just felt different; he felt different. His wife was supportive, but even she was struggling with his negativity. He just couldn't get out
of his head the notion that here he was, at what he felt ought to be something
like the prime of his life, and in fact all he could think about was the possibility of
a future as a cripple. Not a very politically correct word, he knew, but for him
that was his stark reality. And he couldn't face it, didn't want to face it, and
didn't know what the hell to do about it. He knew there were horrible diseases
around affecting mobility, and he tried to put it out of his mind, but . . .

'So. I don't know how much you've talked about what's happening to you, Gerry,
but I want to offer you this counselling time to talk it through, or whatever is on
your mind.'

Gerry nodded. He didn't know what to say. He'd talked to his wife, and she was
good, but somehow he didn't feel able to talk to her about how he really felt.
He kind of felt he wanted to protect her from that. But he also knew that he
wasn't handling it too well. Things were tense at home a lot of the time. He sort
of wanted to talk but he didn't want to burden her. Now here he was, with time
to talk to someone, and he didn't know what to say or where to begin.

He had been struck by the fact that Maureen seemed a pleasant enough person
but he wasn't sure about this counselling lark. He didn't see how talking
about his problems to a stranger would help. It was his wife he needed to talk
to but he couldn't, so really he just wanted to learn how to keep his fears to
himself and not let them upset him. He just wanted some hope, but he felt like
no one could give him that. As he sat there, there was a pain in his head behind
his eyes and his legs were tingling, kind of pins and needles. It seemed to come
and go, but he didn't really understand why. He just never really knew from
day to day, although in a way he did. When it was bad it lasted for a while;
it was more a case of never knowing when a run of 'good' days would end.

'I don't know where to begin, really. I mean, it's been a real shock and I guess I haven't been handling it too well. The GPs referred me to the neurologist for tests. He hasn't said what he thinks is happening.'

Maureen nodded. 'Yes, Dr Ahmed mentioned it in his referral letter. He also told me that you have been referred to the consultant neurologist and were awaiting an outpatient appointment.'

> The counsellor makes it clearly visible what is in the referral letter. This ensures transparency. The client now knows what the counsellor is aware of, although, of course, she has received it from the perspective of the GP.

Gerry nodded. 'He thought I should see you because, well, he said I seemed depressed. Said he didn't want to put me on any medication, not at this stage, said he hoped counselling would help. Said he thought I needed to talk to someone.'

'Yes, he mentioned that. I'm glad he referred you to me first. Sometimes medication is necessary but sometimes talking things through eases the pressure and helps mood to bounce back a little.'

> Depression can have an organic basis and a chemical intervention becomes necessary to lift and stabilise mood. However, depression can also be reactive to circumstances, to life experience. In such instances, anti-depressants can helpfully reduce the depressive symptoms although work will be required to resolve that which is causing the symptoms. The difficulty is that the anti-depressants may create a false experience for the client, affecting their ability to engage with their true feelings as opposed to their chemically affected feelings, making it difficult for them to engage with therapy, or indeed feel motivated to do so.
>
> Where depression is deep although the cause is environmental or the result of traumatic life experience, the stabilising effect may be necessary to enable the client to cope with their psychological distress and to help them begin the therapeutic process.

'Yeah, he's put me on some stuff to try and ease the discomfort. Sort of works a bit some days, but not all the time.'

'Mhmm. So the medication doesn't always make a difference?'

'No.' That was one of the things that worried Gerry. He knew how some of these neurological conditions could be progressive, and the fact that the medication didn't always make a difference was alarming him.

Maureen noticed how unhappy Gerry looked, and how worried. She let him know that she was experiencing this.

'It certainly leaves you looking unhappy and worried – I guess that's how it must be?'

Gerry nodded. 'Understatement that. I guess I'll get by.' He knew he was saying that for himself; he didn't want to say how he really felt. It was too uncomfortable. He knew that he was full of fear and wanted to keep it at bay. It just felt all too overwhelming. He struggled to sound OK about things.

Gerry is incongruent. He is saying one thing but feeling something very different. This will lead to heightened anxiety. The person-centred counsellor, through offering the attitudinal qualities of the core conditions, seeks to offer an opportunity for incongruence to be recognised and made visible, with the hope that the client will begin to be able to accept their reality and integrate the emotional discomfort and mental distress that is present for them.

'Understatement but your feeling is that you'll get by, in spite of it all.'

Yes, thought Gerry, that's what I said but it's not what I feel. He felt desperate. But he daren't let his feelings get the better of him; he just knew that he wouldn't cope at all. He had to keep them under control. He decided to change the subject to his neurology appointment.

'At least I've got my appointment with the neurologist. In six weeks.'

'Bit of a wait, and must leave you with all kinds of thoughts and feelings.' Maureen wanted to keep options open for Gerry to take his own direction. She had noticed his switch of focus and she accepted that he was experiencing a need to do this. She wasn't going to redirect him. She wanted to accept him and allow him to be as he needed to be.

Too right, thought Gerry. Deep down he knew he was afraid of what he was going to be told. He knew what people were like with some of the conditions that affected the central nervous system. Motor neurone disease was the one that terrified him the most, although he knew he had no reason to suspect that, but he just didn't know. He just knew something was wrong and it frightened him. He felt like his body was, well, out of control. The thought of what it might be like for him in the future; he just didn't want to think about it. The GP had tried to reassure him that treatment for these kinds of condition had improved greatly in recent years, and that the progression of any kind of disability, if that was what it was, could be controlled far better, but he hadn't really listened. 'Yeah.' He replied, aware that he had tightened his jaw and his lips after he had spoken.

Maureen nodded. She didn't want to say anything more. Clearly Gerry was struggling; he wasn't finding it easy to talk and she wasn't going to start pressuring him in any way. She had long ago realised that even where there were only a limited number of counselling sessions, it was best to let the client find their own pace, and to trust their own process. She believed strongly that people had within them the capacity to make the best of situations, or at least find ways to gain what they needed from opportunities given to them. She knew not everyone took them, but then she also recognised that often this was because the relational climate wasn't helpful. People don't like to be pushed into something uncomfortable; they don't always want to feel that someone else knows what's best for them. Most people had a bellyful of that in childhood, and often still carried the emotional scars or 'introjects' and 'conditions of worth' as person-centred theory refers to them.

The term 'conditions of worth' applies to the conditioning that is frequently present in childhood, and at other times in life, when a person experiences that their sense of worth is conditional on their doing something, or behaving, in a certain way. The person feels they have to be a certain way to have self-worth. With this come attendant beliefs that there are certain ways that they should not be, as this will negate any sense of self-worth. The person is left experiencing a need to behave in certain ways in order to achieve a sense of self-worth. 'Introjects' are beliefs that the person has about themselves. They have been described in person-centred theory as 'an evaluation taken in from the outside and symbolised as defining a dimension of the Self' (Mearns and Thorne, 2000, p. 108). The person seeks to live according to these introjects   for instance, beliefs such as: I am successful, I am a perfectionist, I am useless, I am unlovable, I feel warmth for everyone. But they are difficult to live up to, often offering extremes, and because they are taken in from outside, they are not genuine aspects of the person. People may carry conflicting introjects, leaving them doomed to fail at one whenever they achieve the other.

'This is a tough time to talk about things, Gerry, and I'm not going to push you on anything. I just want to acknowledge what a bloody tough time it must be.'

Gerry looked up and met Maureen's gaze. They sat for what was only a few moments, and yet seemed to Gerry much longer, holding eye contact. There was something about the way that Maureen looked at him. She seemed, well, he kind of felt that she seemed to sort of understand, and yet, how could she? How could she? He was puzzled, but it had felt good. He felt different somehow, more accepting of himself in that moment. Here was a reassurance emerging from somewhere deep within himself and yet, why? He wasn't sure and as he thought about it the experience faded. The moment had passed now, but somehow it had made him feel a little stronger, a little more . . . he didn't know how else to describe it, but something felt different.

Maureen had felt clear and comfortable in that silence. It had felt very real, very important and she had felt very present. It felt to her like something important had happened, some kind of connection had been made, although she didn't feel in a position to define it. However, the moment had passed and she needed to let it go in order to stay with Gerry.

In therapy there are moments of deeper contact when underlying processes seem to be at work, which may not be fully understood by the individual. The effective counsellor can sense these moments and connect with the client in some way – verbally or non-verbally – and something shifts. Movement occurs in these moments. There is a shift of perception in the client. They are opened up perhaps to a wider view of themselves and the flow of experiencing that passes through their field of awareness.

The person-centred counsellor will hope to catch these moments and be fully present for and with the client within the therapeutic relationship when they occur. It is a time at which accurate empathy and authenticity are crucially important. In a way, they may be seen to be akin to the big points in a tennis match: the ones that really need to be won. The very best players raise their game in those points. The best counsellors raise their presence when these moments occur in therapy.

'I-er-I guess I don't know what to say.'

Maureen nodded. 'Mhmm. Difficult, yeah?' She sought to empathise with the difficulty.

Gerry didn't know where to start. So much in his head; he could feel his heart was beginning to thump as well. His throat had gone dry. 'Have you any water?'

'Sure, I'll get some.' Maureen went out to the water dispenser. Dammit, she thought, keep meaning to make sure there are water cups filled and in the room. It had been a rush after the previous client, having to write up the notes and think through a letter to the GP as the client had now ended her run of counselling sessions. It had slipped her mind.

Gerry sat in the room alone, wondering what to do, what to say, how to say it. He got up and moved around a bit; sometimes it helped to ease the sensations in his legs. On this occasion it didn't. He took a deep breath and looked up at the ceiling. 'Why me?' The question hung heavily for him. It was a question he had asked over and over again. It just didn't seem fair. It wasn't fair. He heard himself say the question out loud, just as Maureen came back in with the water. He turned and immediately felt the need to apologise. 'Sorry, I needed to get up and try and ease things off a bit; sitting for too long just means I stiffen up.'

'Do what you need to do, Gerry. Is the seat OK?'

'Yes, thanks, it's me anyway, not the seat.'

'Yeah, but sometimes sitting at different heights, different angles can make a difference.'

'No, I'm OK. Thanks for the water.' Gerry sat back down and drank from the plastic cup. 'These water dispensers are everywhere these days.'

'Yes, maybe they encourage people to drink more water. Which is no bad thing.'

'I don't drink enough water, I'm sure.' Gerry lapsed into silence.

Maureen was aware that this was small talk. She went with it, accepting Gerry's need to say what he was saying. She took a sip from the cup of water she had brought for herself and put it down. It felt like it had been a kind of interval, a sort of halfway break in proceedings. She had glanced at her watch on the way to the drinks machine – halfway through the session. She decided to voice what had been her thinking, wanting to be present to Gerry and to open up the conversation

'As I went out for the water, it felt a bit like an interval, a kind of drinks break mid-session. So I know I'm wondering how you want to use the rest of time we have today.' This was spoken from a genuine experience of thinking about what Gerry might want to use the time for.

Gerry took a deep breath. 'I've got to start talking to someone. I'm bottling too much up. But I don't know where to start.'

'Things you need, want to say, but, yeah, as you say, where do you start. Where do you start ...' Maureen paused and Gerry did not respond. She wondered what was going through Gerry's mind, what was it he wanted to say most but couldn't. 'I'm aware of wondering what are the thoughts and the feelings that can't make it into words.'

Gerry swallowed; his mouth was dry and he took another sip of water. 'I don't know what to do, Maureen – is it OK if I call you Maureen?'

'Sure.'

'I don't know what to do. I started to read up a bit on different neurological conditions. It scared the hell out of me. There are some horrible diseases and it seems there's often no real cure, there can be a sort of containment, symptoms can be managed, it can go into remission, but it's all so problematic.' Gerry went silent. His symptoms, as he had experienced them, seemed to him to be all too close to what he had read about the early onset of multiple sclerosis (MS). He knew that it was preying on his mind. The headaches, the shooting sensations he occasionally got in his back and legs, his struggle to co-ordinate movement sometimes. He'd had some of these symptoms for some while, but had always just regarded them as just a bit of discomfort, too much sitting down, not enough exercise, spending too much time looking at computer screens. He'd had blurry vision for a while. He spoke quietly. 'The doctor won't agree with me, says I need tests, but I think it's MS.' He breathed in deeply and let the air out with a heavy sigh. 'It scares the hell out of me, Maureen, but the symptoms fit, and I know what effect that has on people. I've seen it. Oh God, it scares the hell out of me.'

Maureen took a deep breath. 'Yeah, horrible to think about it. Every reason to scare the hell out of you.' Maureen consciously stayed with Gerry's feelings.

Gerry sat in silence. He was looking down. He felt he needed to reach out to someone, something. It felt too big, too overwhelming, like it just seemed that nothing else was important. All he could think about most of the time – when he didn't have something else to really focus on – was what was happening to his body and what his future would be like. And he didn't like the answers that were in his head.

Maureen stayed with the silence, not wanting to disturb whatever was happening for Gerry. Counselling, for her, was about providing a therapeutic space in which a client could be themselves. In a way, it made more sense to say 'be with themselves', but that kind of suggested a sort of splitting. She wanted Gerry to be able to risk being what was present for him in relationship with her. Seconds passed. Gerry was still looking down.

Gerry lifted his right hand to his face, supporting his elbow with his left hand. He rubbed his eyes with his fingers and thumb and took a deep breath. He could feel his eyes wanting to water but he wasn't going to let that happen. He tightened his jaw and tried to shift his thoughts to something else. He tried to think of his children, of Darius who had recently had a birthday and how happy he had been with his new bicycle. Immediately the thought came in – *but I'll never go on cycle rides with him now.* As a boy he'd loved to cycle, and had been looking forward to sharing that with his son now that he was older. They'd agreed on the bike some while back, before the symptoms had got worse and he'd had to go to the doctor. An offer in a local shop. His brother had kept it at his place – he had space to hide it.

Maureen watched Gerry sitting with his hand over his face, and she noticed him jerk. She realised that he was struggling to stem the tears that were trying to emerge.

'So many tears to express, so hard to let them out.' Maureen spoke from experience and from a genuine sense of what she was observing in Gerry.

Although he hadn't said anything to make it appear that she was offering an empathic response, she was providing an empathic appreciation of the difficulty of expressing painful emotions. She knew that clients didn't necessarily always want empathic *understanding*, that there was a role for empathic *appreciation* of what a client was experiencing, going through, struggling with. Counsellors may not always understand, but they can still convey an appreciation of what they sense to be present for the client.

As he heard her speak, Gerry tightened his eyes. His throat was very dry; he had lowered his hand over his mouth, his eyes still tightly shut. He didn't dare open them. It felt like he would burst, explode, if he opened them. Somewhere he found the strength to quell the tide of emotion and took a deep breath. He took another. 'It's not easy.'

'No.'

'It just seems so bloody unfair.' Gerry emphasised the last two words.

'Yeah, bloody unfair.' Maureen spoke with an edge to her voice, conveying something of the tone that she was hearing from Gerry.

'Why me?'

Maureen took a breath. 'Why me?' Maureen kept with the straight reflection in the first person, and again she reflected in her tone the frustration and despair she could hear in Gerry's voice.

'I just don't know what to look forward to any more.' He paused. The truth was simple and he voiced it. 'I'm not looking forward at all.'

'Hmm. Nothing to look forward to, no reason to look ahead.'

'I can't. I don't know what it'll be like. I've realised how many things I was kind of planning and expecting to do, you know, not that I was thinking about them all the time, but kind of, yeah, dreams and, well, expectations . . .' His voice trailed off.

'Yeah, must feel like they've been swept away – plans, dreams, expectations . . .'

Gerry was shaking his head. 'It's like I've got, well, I mean, I've got a future but I can't see it.'

'Mhmm, know there's a future for you . . .' As she spoke these words she could hear the voice in her head say 'don't want to see it', but that wasn't what Gerry was saying. She stayed with him: '. . . but you just can't see it.'

He shook his head. 'Can't see it, don't want to see it.'

'Yeah.' Maureen nodded, aware she was leaning forward a little more. 'Bit of both, can't see it, don't want to see it.'

'No.' Gerry went silent, at least outwardly. Inside himself he was anything but silent. Going out with his son, going for bike rides, maybe getting him to join a cycle club like he had done when he was younger, all that was gone now.

Maureen was experiencing a really strong urge to ask Gerry what it was that he couldn't or didn't want to see. She was in two minds. She didn't want to push him and direct him, but the question was very present for her. Is this simply my own curiosity, she asked herself. Who am I asking the question for? Gerry knows what he's avoiding thinking about and he's choosing not to tell me. She realised she needed to accept his wish, give him the time and the space to be with what was present for him and let him say what he wanted to say, and wanted her to hear.

Questions can come to mind during a counselling session. The person-centred counsellor will not simply voice what is present for them. They will seek an appreciation of why the question is arising and for whose benefit. As in this instance, Maureen recognises that Gerry will know what he doesn't want to face. She doesn't feel he needs her help to recognise this. She chooses to respect his current decision not to tell her, whatever the reason might be. Rather, she empathises with the difficulty.

'I really want to acknowledge my own sense of how difficult it is to talk about or even think about things that are just too damn painful to be close to.'

Yes, thought Gerry, yes, that's how it is. But he couldn't bring himself to say anything further. He wasn't really aware that he was nodding, ever so slightly.

In a sense Maureen is communicating with that part of Gerry that is remaining silent outwardly but which is very present inwardly. She conveys an appreciation of the kind of difficult process that is present with Gerry, and that part of Gerry which is experiencing this acknowledges it, but it is an acknowledgement to himself, not to the counsellor. This is his struggle. He can acknowledge his fears, his pain, to himself, but making it visible to another is something else.

Maureen noticed that Gerry had nodded in response to what she had said. He was hearing what she was saying and clearly it was connecting with his own internal experiencing. She again allowed Gerry to be with what he was experiencing. He knew how painful it was and she knew that the session was going to have to draw to a close soon. She didn't want that to obstruct his process, but she also wanted him to be aware of the time factor.

'I'm aware we have about ten minutes of today's session left, Gerry. Just wanted you to know in case you've lost track of time.'

Gerry had. In one sense it felt like the session had been an age, and in another way felt like it had been too quick. He suddenly felt a panic. He wanted to say more, but he couldn't. His heart was thumping again. The bicycle, his son, his job, his home, his marriage, his ... his ... freedom. Thoughts rushed in on him and he didn't know what to do with them all. Questions, so many questions. What would he do? How could he carry on? Wheelchair. He pushed that image away, but it was still there. That was his biggest fear, being in a wheelchair, being dependent on others, being imprisoned in a wheelchair. He could feel himself going cold at the thought of it.

'I-I'm ... Oh God, it's the wheelchair, the thought of being in a wheelchair.' He looked up and again met Maureen's gaze. Again the eye contact was held. Maureen held it, staying with the tremendous surge of feeling that ripped through her. Compassion, fear, a wanting to take Gerry in her arms and give him a big hug, and a calm steadiness as well that seemed to emerge from within her as she sat holding eye contact with him. She knew it was more than eye contact. This was psychological contact, full blown, a sharing of a moment, of a client's utter fear and being able to look him in the eye in the midst of his anguish and despair.

Maureen said nothing; the communication was occurring. She had nothing to say. What was there to say? That was Gerry's big fear. Yes. She'd heard it. She felt he knew she had heard it. Words would just break them out of what was occurring between them.

The fact that Maureen had held his eye contact meant so much. Even his wife had struggled, and he hadn't said to her anything about his fear of being in a wheelchair. It had discouraged him from saying more to her. But Maureen seemed to be able to take it, to be there. The moment passed and a little voice in his head started saying, 'Well, she would be like this, she's a counsellor, it's what she's paid to do.' He didn't want to hear it. No, he thought, this felt more than that. But he couldn't put the experience into words. He simply said, 'Thank you.'

Maureen nodded. She wasn't going to ask anything. She accepted what he said by nodding, still holding eye contact.

'OK, so, where do we go from here?' Gerry was thinking about the future sessions.

'In terms of ... ?'

'I was thinking about sessions. Weekly is a bit difficult with work but I'd like to come back next week. How late can you see people?'

'I'm here between 2.00pm and 6.30pm.' Maureen had reached for her appointment sheet. 'I could fit you in with a 5.30pm appointment, but not next week. I'm already seeing someone then, but after that I can go with 5.30pm.'

'OK, I can work something out for next week – what time?'

'It will have to be 3.00pm again.'

'OK, I'll sort that out. I really appreciate the session today although I didn't really say much. But it's been helpful. I feel kind of different somehow, not sure what that's about though.'

'I think it's courageous to start to begin to talk about what's happening for you, your fears, your feelings. It can be *so* intense and overwhelming.' Maureen took a deep breath herself. 'Take care of yourself the rest of the day. It can feel a bit disorientating sometimes for some people.'

'I can believe that. I feel like I have things to think about, and I'll see you next week.' Gerry stood up and reached out his hand. Maureen took it and they shook hands. Again the eye contact was steady. For Maureen it felt like a kind of affirmation of the connection that had been made during the session. For Gerry, well, it was a habit reaction, it's what he always did at work after a meeting with someone. He just did it automatically.

Physical contact at the end of a session can be another moment of powerful communication. It can be the first physical contact, and it could be associated with a moment of eye contact, of communication between two people or it can be a habitual, routine transition action at the end of a period of, in this case, therapeutic contact. The person-centred counsellor will want to be open to their own experiencing of that moment as fully as possible. It is often the last moment of therapy for that client and can leave them with a powerful impression about their therapist.

As he left he was aware of feeling strangely calmer than before the session. Yet he had felt very emotional and upset, though he felt he'd controlled it. But he did feel odd as well. Like he was in a kind of bubble, a bit insulated from the world. Disorientated, that was what she had said. Yes, that was how it felt. He blinked and felt he needed to shake his head. He drove off to the other end of the village where he lived. He was passing the Queen's Arms. He hadn't planned to go back to work that afternoon. He thought he'd drop in for a quick pint. Yeah, felt like that was a good place to sit and think for a while. The kids would be home from school any time and he felt he needed somewhere to, well, just be.

Maureen had written her notes and was making a cup of tea. She had a longer break mid-session, before seeing her final two clients. She found she needed that to catch up on things, but also for herself. She had typed up her letter to Dr Ahmed and decided to take her tea outside. The sun was shining and she felt she needed some fresh air. She was aware that Gerry was still on her mind. It had felt a really intense session. She really had felt a connection even though it had been such a difficult and painful experience for Gerry. She felt in awe of him, of what he was having to come to terms with, the not knowing and yet the sense of knowing what was happening. Yes, the symptoms sounded very

MS-like. She hoped it was some passing problem that would clear itself. And she knew as well that this thought could also be for her own well-being. No, she thought, I can hope that for him, but I have to be open to the experience that he is going to bring of it not being something that will pass, that he is facing the prospect of a long, painful and debilitating progressive disability. She took a deep breath. This was going to be tough and she was sure she'd be using her supervision for exploring and clearing her own reactions.

She had taken a few sips of tea and realised her train of thought had shifted. She realised that she didn't have any particular expectations for the sessions ahead, or any goals. It was the way she worked: get into therapeutic relationship and stay there. Gerry needed someone to listen, try and understand, stay with him on this awful emotional – well, mental and physical as well, and maybe spiritual – journey. Stay with him, be a human being with him, that was her motto. Her clients seemed to benefit from it, if the reduced contacts with the GPs, the reduced use of mood-altering medication and the appreciative comments on the feedback sheets were anything to go by.

Counselling session 2: emotion released and positive ideas

Gerry was sitting in the waiting room; he was a little early again. He had found the first counselling session pretty difficult. It had been a struggle and he was aware that he was holding back. He was pleased that he had managed to mention his fear of being in a wheelchair towards the end of the session. That fear had remained with him after the session. It really sat heavy in the pit of his stomach, and with it came a whole host of other anxieties – would he work, money, his marriage, everything. He'd ended up in the pub longer than he had planned, and drank a little more than he had anticipated. A couple of pints, and they had felt good, had made him feel a little easier somehow. He'd dropped off at the off-licence on the way home and had bought some more beers for the evening.

Maureen came out to call him in. Gerry got up a little unsteadily. It was another bad day, but he was determined to attend. Something in him seemed to be telling him it was important although another part of him didn't want to bother.

'How are things? Another bad day?' Maureen asked the direct question – wanting to connect with Gerry and, while she knew this was directive, it seemed more real to begin this way. Gerry was walking stiffly.

He nodded. 'Yeah.' They entered the counselling room and sat down.

'So, how do you want to use the time we have today, Gerry, anything in particular, anything from last week?' Maureen wanted to keep it open for Gerry to take his own direction.

'It's been a difficult week in many ways. And yet I did feel good about being here last week, even though I found it hard, and it took me a while to get myself together. Dropped off for a couple of beers on the way home – made me feel a little easier.'

'Mhmm, felt good about the session even though it was hard going, but those couple of drinks made it a little easier. And then a difficult week to follow.'

Gerry was nodding. It kind of felt strange hearing what he had said coming back to him. But that was how it had been and hearing Maureen speak somehow focused his attention on how difficult the week had been.

Reordering what the client has said can run the risk of directing the client, often to the last thing that the counsellor says. Best to keep the order as given by the client if you want to be non-directive. It matches their own flow of thinking and feeling, leaving them where they had ended when they were speaking, enabling them to resume from that focus.

'A lot of pain, and not much sleep. I've been tired for a while now, always thought of it as probably work-related, or simply because I wasn't getting enough sleep. Just felt so bloody irritable all the time. Went to work. I don't want to lose that. I can see a day will come when maybe I won't get there, but not now, not yet. There is a part of me that would like to give up, but I know that's not the answer. But it is such a struggle, not just physically. I just don't feel like I have the mental energy either, but I feel I have to keep going. But it takes it out of me. And then I'm not much fun at home, you know?'

Maureen nodded. 'Yes, all the effort, the pain, the tiredness, take their toll on you and at home.'

'I mean, I was thinking after our last session. While I was sitting in the pub, just thinking things through. I don't know, I just kind of felt that I had to get my act together somehow.'

'Mhmm.'

'But when I got home, well, I didn't do much. Had a few beers in the evening and went to bed. Felt horrible the next day. My feet and lower legs were tingling. Don't know why. Never do know really how I'll be until I wake up.'

'So you realised you had to get your act together, but didn't do much when you got home.'

'Just didn't feel like it. Maybe the beers had got to me, I don't know. It does make me feel a bit more relaxed somehow. But it's not the answer. I think I could drown myself in my sorrows if I'm not careful.' He shook his head. 'That's no answer, but it does make me feel easier.'

'Drown yourself in your sorrows and let the beers make it all feel a little easier. And part of you knows that's not the answer.' Maureen was experiencing concern as to how much Gerry might be using alcohol to cope with his feelings, and whether that was playing a part in his depression. But she put the thought aside for the moment.

> A counsellor may be experiencing genuine concern for choices that a client is making; however, the person-centred counsellor will want to respect the client's choices and needs as they perceive them to be. Persistent concern that interrupts the therapist's empathic effectiveness will need addressing, voicing in the session if it is genuinely blocking the relationship, and/or in supervision if it is recognised as being strongly present but is not voiced. The person-centred counsellor is likely to err on the side of voicing these experiences because of the importance to them of transparency, unless they are clear that what is present for them is very much rooted in a particular experience of their own and does not seem related to what the client is saying.

Gerry stretched his back, which was also feeling a bit stiff. 'I'm still asking "why me?", and I don't get any answer.' As he said this he felt partly resigned to it all but also angry as well. It just wasn't fair. It wasn't fair.

'That "why me?" question, you'd really like an answer.'

Gerry took a deep breath and sighed. 'Yeah, and I know there isn't one. I guess I'm carrying some genetic whatever they're called and, well, here I am. Bloody hell.' He shook his head. 'Never believed this would happen to me. I mean, you don't, do you, well, not unless maybe someone in your family has it. But no one has it in my family. My sister, she's fine, really healthy. My parents, neither of them, although my father gets a bit of rheumatism now and then, but he is nearly 70. Look at me. Only in my thirties and already struggling with it. You know, some days I can hardly get hold of a pen, my fingers tingle and I just can't sort of be sure of my grip. I keep taking the tablets. They take the edge off it some of the time, but then I'll go and do something, forget myself and seems like I overdo it and the symptoms get worse. I used to play football, right wing. Hard to believe now. I had a bloody good right foot. And now, some days I have difficulty getting up out of bed.' He took another deep breath and stretched his back again.

Maureen listened attentively to what Gerry was saying. She heard the despair in his voice and felt the heaviness of mood that was present. 'Just about sums it up, hard to get out of bed. And it leaves you bloody angry.'

'More despair than anger, though that's there as well. I don't know.' Gerry was shaking his head again. 'I look back over my life. Funny the things you think about. I wonder sometimes what it's all about. I just took it for granted, you know, being healthy. I mean, you don't think about it, do you?'

'I guess not.'

'I do now, but it's too late.' He sighed again. 'What's the point?'

Maureen responded, 'Yes, that's how it feels now, what's the point.'

Gerry felt awful. Life seemed hopeless. He thought back to Darius's bike. That just seemed to be with him so much, seemed to sum up his frustration, and his sadness. Tears welled up and he couldn't stop them. He was surprised by the forcefulness of the feelings that were suddenly upon him. He lifted his hand to his face. Even crying was painful. Made his headache worse. I can't even fucking cry without it hurting, he thought to himself. So many things he had assumed he would do, and now? Now he didn't know what he'd be able to do. Didn't have a clue. The tears kept flowing, his eyes felt as though they were burning and his throat was very dry, felt like a huge dry lump at the back. He tried to swallow but it didn't make a difference.

'Have some water, Gerry.' Maureen had poured some out before the start of the session and handed the cup to him.

He nodded and said thanks, took a few sips and put it down. Another surge of emotion rose up within him. He wasn't thinking any more, he was just feeling, lost in a world of . . . He couldn't describe it and wasn't trying. He just was as he felt, and he felt terrible: sad, terrified, desperate. It seemed like every part of him was hurting, just one big glob of pain, that's how it felt, and he hated it. Hated himself. Hated everything.

Maureen said nothing for a moment but stayed with her attention focused on Gerry. She was leaning a little forward in her chair, her hands folded in her lap. For some reason the thought flipped into her head that she must look so much like a counsellor. She pushed it away. It felt awkward. She felt awkward, but she didn't know why. She wasn't usually disturbed like this when a client was upset. She wasn't sure what it was about, but it remained with her.

Maureen is attributing her awkwardness to her posture as a counsellor. It could have a different origin, but this is how she has made sense of it and she does not feel it is significant, and it is therefore not made visible to Gerry. Perhaps she might have leaned over, maybe rubbed his upper back, but asking him first that this what she was offering as she might be planning to touch him in an area that is giving him pain. In moments of such despair, the counsellor's reaching out physically can have so much therapeutic value, much more than words can often convey. Maureen has missed a moment of opportunity, perhaps.

Gerry suddenly coughed and it took her attention away from her own feeling of awkwardness. He swallowed, and took some more water.

'I'm sorry. It just gets to me.'

Maureen nodded. 'Do you cry often?'

'Sometimes, when I'm on my own. I feel ashamed. I don't want anyone to see me like this. Certainly not my family. I haven't cried like that in front of anyone, well, probably ever.' He sat back in the chair and looked towards the top of the wall opposite. He noticed that the paint was peeling. His back was stiff again. He tried to free it off by moving a little in the chair. 'Sorry, I'm feeling stiff today. Spent too long yesterday reading through a report at work, leaning forward at my desk. I think that set it off. Must have been sitting awkwardly. And then I didn't sleep good last night, couldn't settle. Thoughts running through my head. Feeling anxious about coming here again. Wondering if I could phone up with an excuse. But I knew that wasn't the answer.'

Maureen noted that he had changed the focus away from his upset. She sensed there was a link. She didn't want to make it, but chose rather to empathise with what Gerry had been saying. 'It's really awful, feeling ashamed. And you thought about not coming today, but . . .' She left the sentence unfinished, not feeling too sure what to say herself. That awkwardness was back with her again. It had blocked her empathic sensitivity. She wasn't sure what to do with it. She thought about saying it, but felt that somehow the therapeutic relationship she had with Gerry hadn't really developed enough for that. Or had it? She realised she was now embroiled in her own thinking, and she wasn't focused on Gerry. She brought her attention back to him.

Gerry just sat there; he suddenly felt empty. Felt like he had no energy left. He felt heavy in the chair. He had his head back against the back of the chair and he closed his eyes for a moment. It felt a relief, somehow, and made him realise just how tired he was. He could feel his heart pounding away in his chest but he felt strangely calm. He was amazed at the range of feelings he was experiencing. Counselling! Bloody hell, he thought, what a rollercoaster. He didn't want to open his eyes, he just wanted to drift off, escape, fly away into some beautiful place where there was no pain, where he could move freely again and just . . . the word that came to mind was *float*. Yes, he thought, if I could just float away, wouldn't that be wonderful. He was totally absorbed in his world of dreams.

Maureen had watched his head go back and saw him close his eyes. Saw him take a deep breath and let it out, his chest rising and falling. Gradually his breathing had got lighter. His facial expression had changed; he was almost smiling. It made him look younger, somehow.

Maureen is allowing Gerry to be as he feels he needs to be. No external introjects coming from Maureen to imply he must behave in a certain way. There is an openness and acceptance being communicated. It can help to validate, for Gerry, the acceptability of his own needs, and of his meeting those needs for himself.

A sharp twinge of pain in his lower back brought Gerry back. He opened his eyes, somewhat reluctantly. He rubbed his lumbar region, not that it made any difference. 'Sorry.'

'No need to be sorry on my account. You actually looked like you were sort of at peace there, you were smiling.'

Gerry smiled again. 'I just came over feeling so tired. I closed my eyes and then, well, I just felt like I wanted to float away, and I kind of did, so to speak. And then my back reminded me of the real world and brought me back with a thump. Just get this shooting pain.'

'Rude awakening. You'd like to close your eyes and float away from it all?'

He nodded. 'They say exercise is good for you, don't they, and I've heard that people can find it helpful to go into water. I wasn't thinking of water just then, more about floating off into the air, but maybe I should try that.'

Maureen nodded. 'Float about in water?'

'And maybe take some gentle exercise. What do you think?'

Maureen really wanted Gerry to make his own decision, but he had asked a direct question, although she had no idea herself whether or not hydrotherapy could have benefits for people with MS. It made some sense though, keep the muscles active, maybe it would help. But she really didn't know. However, she didn't want to discourage Gerry. 'Sounds good. How does the idea feel to you?'

'I think it would be a good idea. I wouldn't want to go mad, just a bit of gentle exercise. I could take Darius as well, perhaps. Maybe it's something we could do together.'

Maureen felt a real sense of how important that was for Gerry, something deep inside her felt touched as he had said that last sentence. 'Maybe that's something we could do together.' She smiled. She hadn't intended to repeat what Gerry had just said word for word out loud, but she had.

Gerry was suddenly puzzled, and taken aback. She wants to come swimming with me? The look of puzzlement spread across his face and Maureen was unsure what had caused it. She hadn't been thinking about what she had just said.

'You look puzzled?'

Gerry felt awkward, not sure what to say. Had he misheard her? He must have done. He decided to let it go, must have been his mistake. 'No, I thought you said . . . no, never mind. I must have misheard you.'

Maureen was now trying to think back. Oh shit, she realised what she must have said. 'I was reflecting back what you had said, you know, you and your son going swimming together.' She suddenly felt a little embarrassed.

Gerry's face broke into a broad grin. 'I thought, oh what an idiot, I thought you were offering to come swimming too!' He began to laugh; so did Maureen.

'Nice thought, but I don't tend to go swimming with my clients!' Shit, that felt a bit flirty, she thought straight away. Something for supervision.

'No, I'm sure you don't.' Gerry was still smiling and somehow a tension had eased in the room.

Maureen noticed it too. She wondered if it had all been so heavy and serious and perhaps a moment of light relief had somehow shifted them both. Maybe they both needed it. Well, it's happened now. She wasn't averse to humour in sessions. Sometimes it could bring people together, bring out a different facet of the common humanity between client and counsellor.

> Humour does play an important part in the therapeutic process. It can pro-
> vide for intimate moments of psychological contact, a mutual sharing of a
> perception on something. It can bring together.
>
> Yes, it can be a way of avoiding something painful as well, but that's OK.
> It is a legitimate choice. The person-centred counsellor trusts the client to
> know how they need to be and will seek to be warmly accepting of them.
>
> Humour can also sometimes reflect a shift of perspective, expressive of the
> client discovering perhaps a sense of the ridiculous towards some event that
> had previously been so deadly serious. It can be indicative of their opening
> up to a fuller range of experience in relation to something. It can help dis-
> solve – or perhaps it is a sign of the dissolution of – a certain rigidity.

Maureen decided to bring the focus back. 'So, you think it would be a good idea to
take some exercise in water and take your son along as well?'

'Yes. I know he likes swimming. I'll see what he says.'

'I hope it helps.'

'So do I. At least it's maybe something we can do together. I'll have to take it
easily, don't want to overdo it. Guess I'll have to explain it to him a bit. I can
do that. He's going to realise sooner or later, if he hasn't already.' Gerry felt a
little more positive all of a sudden. Yes, something to look forward to, something to do, somewhere to go with Darius. He'd check it out. He wasn't sure
when, but maybe at the weekend. He felt it would be too much in the week
and anyway Darius had homework. Yes, he'd check out the hotel nearby that
had a health club, see what the membership was. He'd do it on the way home.

'Yes, that's true, and maybe you want to tell him yourself in your own way?'
Maureen realised that her reply wasn't empathic, just a conversational sugges-
tion. Somehow the session had moved into conversation. She decided to go
with it. It seemed OK.

Gerry nodded. 'Yes, but I think I may need to tell them both together. I think I
need to do that. They must have noticed that I'm not so active these days, at
least I don't move so freely. I need to talk to Carol about it, but, yes, I do need
to talk to them. Somehow I kind of know it's MS. Too many matching symptoms.' Gerry paused. Yes, he thought, I'm sure that's what it is, the shooting
pains, the headaches, the sensations in his feet and legs, the blurred vision.
He took a deep breath. 'Funny. It feels in a way a huge thing to do, and yet it
doesn't as well. It's like, I know I have to tell them. And it'll be OK, somehow.
But I don't want to worry them. I want to reassure them that everything will be
OK, but I'm just going to have to take things a little easier.'

'That sounds important to you, reassuring them. I think it will be a big step,
Gerry, and an important one.'

'Yes. Maybe it will be good for me to talk to them. I haven't so far, not really, but
talking here, well, I've survived the ordeal, haven't I? No, seriously, thanks for
listening and letting me talk. I seem to have found some kind of reassurance

for myself from somewhere, and I can't explain from where. But I think I can talk to them now. I'm not going to get upset. I know that. I just need to tell them. They're bright kids. I'll make sure that I combine it with a treat of some kind.' Yes, that felt the right thing to do.

Maureen was feeling a sense common to her, that of amazement as to how people could change simply by talking, and feeling listened to and heard. However much she believed in each individual's potential to discover inner resources to overcome difficulties or to find ways of moving through difficult experiences, and the role that creating a therapeutic relationship had in facilitating this, she still wondered at it.

'Mhmm. Sounds like you're already beginning to plan it.'

'Yes, they've been wanting to go to the fun fair and, well, bank holiday is coming up next weekend, so, yes, I'll have a chat to them. I guess it'll be a case of sitting round the table. Family meal times. Always hated them as a kid, always wanted to get away and do my own stuff. Never had a TV in the dining room at home. That was a pain. But my parents insisted on it. Didn't think much to it at the time but now, yeah, I'm glad we did that because we carry it on as well. Time together, to talk. I've got some things to talk about, but I think I need to talk to them after I've talked to Carol. I know it has to come from me, but it feels right that it should be from both of us as well.'

'Seems like you are really making a firm decision on this, Gerry. It feels good to me hearing you speak like this.' Maureen wondered whether that had been a helpful comment. She didn't want to convey a sense that she didn't feel good about Gerry speaking when he was feeling low and upset. She felt warmly accepting of him however he needed to be, but she also couldn't deny that she did feel good hearing a positive edge in his voice. It hadn't been much in evidence up until now. But she was concerned as to how Gerry would interpret what she had said.

'I feel good, too. Something positive I can do.'

Maureen nodded. 'You've felt a lot of things this session, and I want to honour them all, and, yes, it is important to have some kind of positive focus, and I realise that there are and will be times when that will seem a million miles away.'

'I know.' Gerry paused. He was suddenly very thoughtful again, not heavy or weighed down, but just feeling very quiet once more. 'I know.'

Maureen nodded and they held eye contact. It was a powerful moment again, just as it had been in the previous session. It felt like Gerry needed that contact, like it somehow held him, reassured him in some way. But she didn't know. Maybe she was reading too much therapy into it.

For Gerry, it did seem somehow powerfully reassuring but he didn't understand why. But Maureen seemed to have a steadiness, a kind of reliance. He was realising more and more that he felt he could trust her. He took a deep breath and looked away towards the clock. The session was coming to an end.

'I don't know what significance eye contact has for you, but I'm aware that it seems important, and the sense I had was something to do with reassurance, but that could be just me.'

Maureen chooses to voice her experience and open up the possibility of further exploration should Gerry wish to do this. She is making visible her feelings, seeking transparency, and thereby encouraging the same in her client.

'You feel steady, someone I can kind of rely on, someone who, I don't know, it's hard to describe, but I do sense that you are listening, really listening, and that feels very important to me at the moment. Sometimes I feel like I'm going mad, but you take me seriously, you listen, you tell me what you hear and what you feel. That feels good, somehow. Like, it sort of feels real? No games.'

Maureen nodded. 'Yeah, no games.' Another moment of connection and a silence. She added, 'None of this is a game.'

Gerry took a deep breath and let it out slowly. 'Yeah, that's for sure.' He tensed himself, getting ready to head off.

The session drew to a close. They agreed to continue with weekly appointments, but at the later time. Maureen asked Gerry whether their sessions would overlap with his appointment with the neurologist, and he said that they would. In fact, he said he was glad she'd mentioned it because the appointment was the same afternoon as that sixth session and he wondered if he could have that one the following week. His appointment was late in the afternoon and he felt he wanted to go home afterwards and talk to his wife, rather than come to counselling that day.

Maureen felt that was positive – she didn't like to feel clients became dependent on counsellors, turning to them rather than to their own loved ones. It was Gerry and Carol who were facing this together. She, Maureen, was the skilled helper, the person that Gerry could explore himself freely with, but it was important to her that he then took what he had gained back into his relationship with Carol. She watched him leave and returned to her seat and spent a few minutes just being quietly with herself, allowing feeling and thoughts to be present spontaneously. She felt positive. She felt that something had shifted for Gerry. That talking and being listened to was helping him to find his voice and want to talk to his family. She was glad, for him and for them. It was an important step and she wanted to really support him in this decision. Only time would tell what effect it would have on him, and on them, of his being open about everything.

And she recognised, too, that things could change again. The future remained uncertain for Gerry; he had a lot of adjustment to make and no doubt a lot of pain to face. She realised that she was feeling a lot of respect for him. Multiple sclerosis is such a silent disease, doesn't grab the headlines like cancer, but it could lead to so many different associated health problems, and to premature death. Like many other progressive disabilities, they can seem somehow less in the headlines – unless someone famous happens to be suffering with it. So many people suffered with disabling conditions. So much pain and misery. Her thoughts went to the consultants who worked with people with these kind of neurological conditions. So many people wasting away, helpless as their bodies began to fail them. How did the specialists maintain their motivation, seeing so much pain and suffering, people struggling to cling to their mobility, their independence? Occasional periods of remission but for so many a gradual decline. What a future for Gerry to have to contemplate, and his wife. How would she bear up? How would he cope? And Maureen knew how important it was for her to be there for and with Gerry over the next few weeks.

Points for discussion

- Assess the impact of Maureen's empathic responding on Gerry.
- What criteria do you use to assess whether an urge to say something in a session should be voiced? How does this relate to person-centred theory?
- What feelings and thoughts are you left with about Gerry, and how might they impact on your work with him if you were his counsellor?
- So much can be conveyed through eye contact. How helpful was it for Maureen to voice her experience?
- How did Maureen convey her warm accepting of Gerry?
- Discuss instances of congruence and incongruence during the session.
- Write your own notes for these two sessions.

CHAPTER 2

Supervision session 1: exploring the counsellor's reactions to her client

Maureen had been talking about some of her other clients in the supervision session and she wanted to spend some time talking about Gerry and the impact on her of working with him.

'I have another new client at the surgery, referred in by the GP. He's experiencing symptoms which he's convinced are of MS though he's waiting to see the neurologist. He's getting shooting pains and headaches, blurred vision, his movement isn't good. Seems he is needing space to talk through coming to terms with it and the implication for his future.'

Donna nodded. 'That sounds quite heavy and I notice from your tone of voice that there's suddenly a real seriousness in the atmosphere.'

'Yes, it's a tough one.'

'Seen other clients in this position?'

Maureen shook her head. 'No, not like this, waiting for a diagnosis with a head full of fears that are just, yeah, what you'd feel.'

'So I'm wondering how it is leaving you feeling and what impact that is having on the forming of the therapeutic relationship. How many times have you seen him?'

'Twice. The first session he really struggled to say much about it. There were a lot of feelings present but he was trying to hold them back. But towards the end he became more emotional and talked about his fear of being in a wheelchair. Said that giving his son a bicycle for his birthday recently had brought home to him how limited he was becoming. So many assumptions about his future are evaporating. A lot of loss.'

'Yeah, and I appreciate that hearing you speak about him there is a real sensitivity coming across to me.'

'I really feel for him, for his struggle to make sense of it and to adjust to it all. I know that remission can occur, but for many people the future is one of pain and disability, and he's only in his early thirties. I know people much younger than him develop the condition, but that's no help to Gerry. He has to find his own way through this.'

'Yes, your head knows that remission can occur but your feelings ...? I'm aware of not hearing about your feelings.'

> The supervisor hasn't heard about the impact on her supervisee's feelings and offers an opportunity to explore this.

'I feel the awesome nature of what he is facing, the huge impact that it is having and will have on his life, you know, I mean, all of his life. I am aware after being with him how much I take my own health for granted in many ways. It's the kind of thing that you think will happen to someone else. You don't think about it in relation to yourself, at least, not unless it is in the family or has affected a close friend and you already have an appreciation of how it can affect people.' Maureen wasn't feeling unduly emotional as she spoke; somehow the hugeness of it all was leaving her feeling, well, she wasn't sure exactly what it was, there was a kind of numbness that sort of seemed linked to the overwhelming nature of it all. She had gone quiet.

'Can feel overwhelming?' Donna was sensing that Maureen was very much in awe of it all. It felt huge.

'It makes me feel somehow quite small. Like where do you begin? I mean, I know I can't make it better, I can't even really offer him hope.'

'It feels hopeless to you?' Donna was interested in pursuing this sense of hopelessness. Was Maureen feeling impoverished, deskilled in some way, she wondered.

'I can only imagine what it must feel like to be faced with something like this.'

Donna nodded. 'It's left to your imagination.'

'And it's hard to connect with what it must feel like.'

'You feel unable to connect with your own feelings?'

> An important question, summing up the difficulty that Maureen is facing. It leaves her exploring in her own mind whether this is so. It also opens her to focus on her own experiences in this area, and a memory surfaces as a result.

The room had gone quiet, and both were talking quietly and reflectively. Maureen thought about that last response. Do I feel unable to connect with *my* feelings? She wondered about it. True, she wasn't sure what she felt. She thought about her own family; no one had had MS. She could remember an aunt who had arthritis and had done for many years. She could remember visiting her as a child. Even then she wasn't too mobile. As a child she hadn't really appreciated it, remembered being told off on one occasion for being too boisterous and running into her aunt, which had caused her pain. She'd been told off about it, but she hadn't really understood why. She'd only been about six or seven at the time. Later on she'd begun to understand. But it had eased for a while in her life, although now she was quite elderly and being cared for in a nursing home. She realised she hadn't seen her for the longest while and made a mental note to do something about that.

'You seem lost in thoughts, Maureen. Anything in particular?'

Maureen smiled. 'I was back in the past.' She told her about the incident with her aunt and how she now realised she wanted to see her, talk to her, maybe try and understand from her what it had been like facing a progressive disability. 'It's not the same, but in her days there weren't the treatments for arthritis that there are today. She has suffered from progressive disability throughout her life. I feel I want to talk to her.'

'Listen to her or say something to her?'

Maureen was back to the incident. She'd felt awful, she'd loved her aunt, and she'd seen her many times later in childhood, but her shriek of pain, she could still hear it. Maureen felt her emotions rising, the tears in her eyes, and they began to seep out and down her cheeks. 'I didn't understand. I didn't mean to hurt her, but I did. They told me off, but I didn't know, I didn't understand.'

Donna sensed the shift and stayed with Maureen. 'You didn't understand, how could you, you were a small child.'

'But they made me think that I should have known, should have understood, should have been more careful.'

'Mhmm, should have known, should have been more careful, but you didn't know.'

'No, I didn't.' Maureen felt the tide of emotion passing, and began to dry her eyes. 'But I needed to.'

'Your need to know sounds quite important to you.'

As Maureen heard Donna she found herself flipping back to Gerry. She shook her head. 'That's it, isn't it? Needed to know, should have known. She hadn't told me about her pain. I should have known. Gerry hasn't really told me about his pain, and again I should know, I need to know. I've got to be careful, here. Stuff from the past, it never lets you go, does it?'

Donna shook her head. 'Can leave us with sensitivities however much we work on it.'

'OK. So, I can see my sensitivity, and I need to be aware of that. I need to be open but allow Gerry to go at his pace. The "should know" from the past I have to ignore. That was then, not now. But I do feel I need more knowledge of Gerry's condition generally. Someone suffering from MS isn't something I've worked with a great deal. Maybe I should contact one of the MS networks, get some information. I don't know, I feel I need to know more. And as soon as I hear myself say that, I know as well that in reality I'm working with feelings of loss, or at least potential loss, which I am used to working with.'

'But there is something different about this?'

Maureen nodded. 'Yes.'

'Can you get hold of what that difference is, what it feels like?' Donna was circling her hands in front of her as she spoke. She could feel inside herself an urge to somehow get some clarity, some sense of what it was that Maureen was experiencing.

Part of the last session came back to her, that feeling of awkwardness that had suddenly arisen in her and persisted for a while. 'There were times in the last session when I felt awkward.'

'Awkward?'

The supervisee has moved to a recognition of a particular feeling that has been present for her in the sessions.

'Yes, a kind of uncomfortable awkwardness. It's kind of difficult to describe, but I felt sort of, well ...' She thought about it more. 'Well, awkward. But there was more to it than that. It was quite strong, you know, and, yes, really uncomfortable.'

'Mhmm, so something about what was happening was leaving you feeling this way, uncomfortable, awkward, and it persisted.'

'Yes.'

'Can you reconnect with that feeling now rather than think about it?' Donna was aware that there could be a tendency in supervision to talk about feelings when often what was needed was an opportunity to connect with them and allow them to become present and experienced in the session. Often that helped the supervisee to process them.

Maureen sat. She was aware she was thinking about them. 'I'm still in my head, here. I need to get into my body, I think.'

Donna was struck by that comment. 'Need to get into your body. Somehow there's a kind of physiological reaction but you're not in touch with it?' She was mindful that Gerry was bringing an issue concerned with emotionally and mentally coming to terms with a physical condition.

Maureen sat and brought herself in her imagination to how it had been with Gerry. She allowed herself to be with the issues he had brought, with his upset, his tears, his despair, his needing an answer to that question, 'Why me?' She could feel a knot in her solar plexus, heavy, dark. Her arms felt strangely numb. She stayed with the experience. She felt heavy in the chair, like it was hard to move. She felt tired; she could feel her eyes getting heavy. There was a kind of bleakness to the experience. A real sense of what's the point. That was what Gerry had said, at least, she thought he had.

'What are you feeling, Maureen? You look very serious.' Maureen had her eyes closed and her face seemed quite tense.

The supervisor offers an opportunity for Maureen to put into words what has become present for her. She is now exploring elements that were present at some level within herself within the session but which, at the time, she was not connected with and which could have affected the quality and nature of her empathy, and certainly her degree of congruence.

'It feels really bleak, and heavy, and a sense of "what's the point?". It feels like I'm surrounded by . . . well, it's like a kind of heavy treacle but it isn't. It's not sticky or anything like that.' She thought about it some more, trying to get a sense of what would describe this feeling, the sensation that was pervading her body. Her mind suddenly thought of how she was sitting on the earth, held down by gravity. She wasn't sure where the image had come from, but it made sense. Yes, gravity. 'I've got it, it feels like gravity has increased, like there's a pull on me, making it difficult to move easily.' She was amazed how heavy she was feeling, yet she knew nothing had changed, not really changed, and yet she felt so heavy, so stuck.

'So there's a real heaviness, like gravity has increased and is sort of pinning you down?'

'Not exactly pinning me down. I know I can move, I know I have that freedom, and yet it's difficult.' She realised she was back to thinking about Gerry. 'I'm back in my head again, thinking about Gerry. The thought has just struck me that as I sit here feeling the heaviness, the difference is that he's in pain, I'm not.'

'Mhmm, he's in pain and you're not.'

'And that . . .' Maureen stopped again, yes that was it. 'Yes, I'm not in pain and he is, and I feel uncomfortable about that.'

'So not sharing his pain, or not being in pain, makes it uncomfortable for you to be with him?'

'If I was in pain like him, maybe it would be easier to listen to him. Not sure why I said that.' Maureen had her eyes closed as she sat trying to stay in touch with the experience.

'Mhmm, if you had his pain, then maybe . . .'

Maureen cut into what Donna was saying. 'Yes, if I had his pain, yes, that's it. That's the awkwardness.' She opened her eyes and was aware that the heaviness was passing and she was suddenly beginning to feel more alert again. 'Yes, I feel awkward because I'm pain-free, he isn't. I feel that I ought to be feeling what he is. It's like, we hear our clients talk about their emotional pain, you know, and we can get a sense of that, sometimes. I mean, we don't actually feel what they feel, but in a way we do, kind of tune in, be somehow in their world, their frame of reference.'

The supervisee makes a connection. She has realised the roots of the awkwardness that she has felt and has, in effect, integrated the experience more fully into her experience. It will enable her to become more fully and authentically present with her client.

Donna was nodding and listening intently, very aware that Maureen had shifted quite clearly from being heavy and serious-looking to being suddenly more alert. She didn't say anything, simply nodded slowly, not wanting to interfere with Maureen's train of thought.

'But this is physical pain as well and I cannot get into that experience. I can get a sense of his despair, his feelings about his pain, and yes, I've had headaches, but ... oh, I don't know, I cannot get into the pain itself. And that's what feels awkward. Like I cannot get into part of his experience.'

'OK, you can't get into his physical pain, but you can sense and feel something of the nature of his emotional pain.'

'Yes, his fear of the future, his sense of loss, yes, those are present. I can relate to them. I can sense their presence. But the physical pain, no, I've not experienced that kind of pain – I mean I've had physical pain, but not what he must be going through.'

'You need to experience his pain, or pain like his, to feel you can empathise?'

'I think I do.'

'Mhmm. It has to be his pain?'

'Not sure what you mean; it sounds like you've something in mind.'

'Well, we don't necessarily experience our client's emotional pain, but our emotional reaction to their pain which is then kind of informed by our own experiences of emotional pain. Does that make sense?'

'Yes. So I can hear and appreciate what my client tells me of their emotional pain, using my experience of my own feelings when I am with them and my own experiences in my own life, yes?'

'Is that making sense in relation to your experience?'

'Yes, it is.' Maureen stopped for a moment, thinking about all of this. OK, so I can use my knowledge and experience of pain to get an appreciation for what a client is going through; we have a kind of emotional language even though I cannot actually really know what my client is feeling from the words they use because they may be attaching a different meaning to the one I do to a particular word. But we have enough to communicate and for me to gain an empathic understanding. 'But I can't get into his physical pain, Donna, I can't get a sense of what it must be like.' She thought back over the sessions. 'I can't remember him really describing the pain, or has he and I've lost it?' She couldn't recall. 'I don't think he has.'

'OK, so he hasn't really talked about it, and you sense a difficulty in actually being able to appreciate what his personal pain is like, and it leaves you with some inner discomfort and an awkwardness.' Donna sought to sum up where they had got to. She was aware that their time was nearly up, but she also sensed that the exploration hadn't ended. But maybe it didn't have an end; it would continue during the time Maureen was working with Gerry. Or maybe it was a simple fact that if you hadn't genuinely experienced a particular physical pain, it was difficult to really empathise with the experience of someone else for whom that pain was a reality.

'I mean, I know pain, the physical pain I've experienced. You don't give birth to children without knowing that, and, yes, I have pain, but it is *my* pain. It's kind of personal to me in some way.'

'Something very personal about physical pain; your pain is not your client's pain.'

'No. I need to be able to get a sense of his pain.'

'Your need?' Donna was aware of the forcefulness of what Maureen had said.

'Hmm, that doesn't sound very person-centred, it's my client's needs that are important, but no, I have a need here as well. I need to appreciate more his pain.' She paused. 'I'm not getting in there. I need to get in there, I need to be more open, somehow. I think I'm closed down. It's no good. I need to be affected. Dammit, I want to be affected.'

'You're fired up, Maureen. What's happening for you?'

'Frustration, despair.' She could feel tears welling up. 'Shit. He's a lovely guy, he's got to me. I want to make it better. I can't. Why do people have to suffer like this? I watched a TV programme last night about someone coping with disability, lost the use of their arms and legs. Talking about their struggle to accept their situation, how they fought against accepting it, battled, argued with God, pleaded, but nothing changed, just got worse.'

'Why do people suffer? And you're suffering as you think about it.'

'Makes me so angry. Just doesn't seem fair. Is this it? One life, and the dice are loaded?'

'Strong feelings, Maureen, how the hell do we make sense of it?'

'I guess everyone has their own way, I just haven't found one.'

'What makes it hard to accept it with Gerry?'

'He's a nice guy, just doesn't seem fair. Guess I warmed to him pretty quickly, think I've got too much sympathy and not enough empathy.'

'Mhmm, that's how it feels?'

'But I care. And yet he hasn't really told me that much about his pain.'

'Maybe he isn't ready yet to tell you, Maureen. As you said earlier, it's personal, it's an intimate experience, maybe he's not ready yet to be that personal.'

Maureen took a deep breath. 'You're right, of course. Yes. Yes. But I still want to get in there.'

Donna nodded. 'Yes, I hear you, and Gerry must decide what he is going to tell you, and when. But perhaps what we have talked about has left you more open in some way to him, and maybe you'll be different in the next session because of this?'

'I think I will. I do feel different, more alert, more present somehow. Something has shifted in me. More aware of my reactions, of what I feel about it all. Yeah, that feels good. I need this. That's partly why I come, of course.' She smiled.

Maureen acknowledges that a shift in her experiencing of herself has occurred. The comment 'more present somehow' is significant. She is becoming more open to the range of reactions that have been occurring within her in response to Gerry. She will feel more present because more of her is present to her. This means that there is a higher likelihood that more of her will be emotionally/psychologically present for Gerry, which in turn will help more of him to come into the therapeutic relationship.

'Yes, part of the mystery of supervision is how we unravel these kinds of knots through this process. But we shouldn't be surprised. It's similar to what clients do when they talk though issues.'

'I know, but I am grateful for it. I learn so much, and it is a constant exploration of myself. I know we talk about clients, but often it comes down to *me*, *my* reactions, *my* process, how *I'm* affected by the client. It's just such a privilege in many ways to have this space.'

'Yes, and a professional requirement, of course, to ensure that we are safe, the client's safe, and that we are really able to be authentically and empathically present in a warm and accepting relationship with our clients.'

'Thanks, Donna.'

The session drew to a close. Maureen felt ready to work with Gerry, somehow more enlivened, more present and ready to connect with him therapeutically and as a human being. Maureen left feeling nourished and enriched by the experience. She realised she was chasing words to hang on her experience. She let it go. She didn't need words. She knew she was in a different place and it felt like the right place to be. It felt healthy. She felt more alive. She turned on the radio, Mendelssohn's Italian Symphony. She breathed in deeply, allowing the sound to permeate her being. It felt good to be alive. And there was Gerry. What did he need at this moment to feel good to be alive?

Counselling session 3: Gerry talks about his emotional sensitivity

'Well, I've talked to the children and it has made it all a lot easier at home. They seemed to take it on board, you know, in fact, they both really seemed to be affected. I was, I know I could feel my eyes watering, and I was kind of glad about that. And that's really strange. There's no way I would have felt OK about that, well, certainly not before coming here. So something has changed in me. I feel more able to accept my emotions, my upset, and it showed.'

Maureen was really pleased for Gerry. It felt like a tremendous achievement and she acknowledged this. 'A big step for you to take, a really big step, and what an affirmation of change as well.'

'Exactly. It felt such a relief. Carol was there, of course, and it seemed to bring us much closer. But it felt such a huge thing to do, to say what my fears were, but that we would face it together and it would be OK. Made me think of the fairy tales we used to have as children – always involved something horrible but it was OK, you could face that because something positive came at the end, though you didn't know it at the time. The kids went out to play and I talked a bit more to Carol. We'd spoken the previous evening and agreed to be open about things with the children. We made it clear nothing was certain, but it was why daddy hadn't been too happy lately. They were great.' Tears welled up in his eyes, and he rubbed them with the back of his hand. It left him blinking, still tearful and feeling very emotional.

Maureen leaned over and took his hand. 'Their reaction . . .'

Gerry was nodding, his eyes screwed up, his lips tight. It had been so important to say something. It was when they'd come over and hugged him, and said they loved him; he'd managed to hold it together, but once they'd gone out he'd collapsed into tears with Carol. It had felt such a release. But it had taken it out of him as well. He'd had to lie down and rest before they went out later. Gerry had taken a couple of tissues and was drying his eyes once again.

'So, I was going to say that was good, but it was so much more than that.'

'Sounds like it was everything.'

'Yeah. It just feels like a huge hurdle. Like I maybe won't bottle things up the same now.' He smiled. 'Anyway, we went out later that day and had some fun and I kind of felt part of the family again.' Gerry could feel emotions rising in him again, and he didn't fight them. He let his eyes water and he felt his throat go dry. 'I guess I'd kind of lost contact with them. So centred on myself, on what was happening for me, you know, I'd moved away from them. I couldn't see it then, but I can now. It feels so much better to be in touch with them again. I can't begin to tell you how important that feels.' He felt a tear trickle down his cheek. He reached for another tissue.

Maureen empathised with his final sentence. 'Hard to really say how important it is, how precious it is.' It felt precious to her; she had the image of a wonderful jewel, shining yet needing to be protected in case it became soiled in some way. 'I've got the image of a precious jewel you want to keep sparkling.'

Gerry was nodding. And smiling, and with tears in his eyes again. 'They're so important to me, Maureen, so important.'

Maureen noted that it was the first time she could recall Gerry calling her by her name. It seemed to fit given the personal and intimate nature of the feelings that Gerry was experiencing in relation to his family, and which he was bringing into the session and sharing with her.

'So, so important.' Maureen spoke slowly and softly, allowing Gerry time to be with the feelings that were connected with his sense of his family's importance to him.

Gerry felt a warmth inside him as he allowed himself to be open to that importance. It had been such a good day; they'd been to the fair and tried different things. The kids had eaten all kinds of stuff and they'd all got back tired but happy, stopping for fish and chips on the way, which the children had both wanted. He'd not only felt part of the family but he had felt like he was a father again, and a husband. Yes, that was strange. He realised he wanted to talk about it to Maureen.

'I had this strange sense that I was feeling like a father again, you know, and a husband. It was like by being with the family and doing things together I kind of found my place again. I hadn't realised I'd lost it, but I can see that I had. I'd lost myself, now I feel I've found myself again.'

'Mhmm, found yourself again as a father and as a husband.'

As he heard Maureen respond he realised he was nodding and he had another realisation break in on him. He added, '. . . and as a man'.

'And as a man.' Maureen responded in the same tone of voice as Gerry had used, steady and with a strong sense of seriousness. She felt that this was a really important realisation. She allowed Gerry time to be with his affirmation.

Maureen conveys her empathy for what Gerry has realised through reflecting his words and tone. The tone conveys her empathic understanding of how important this realisation has been for Gerry. She is taking it seriously, taking him seriously, and conveying respect for something that is important to him.

Gerry hadn't really made the connection until now, but that was what it was really about. Feeling like a man. He shook his head. He was momentarily lost in his own thinking. He'd read about erectile dysfunction as being one of the symptoms or effects associated with MS. He'd not had problems, but it was a concern. He didn't want to talk about that. He came back into his awareness of being in the counselling session, and looked up at Maureen. He brought his thoughts back to what he had been saying. 'Miles away for a moment there.' He thought back to what he had been saying, yeah, hard to feel he was a man. He took a deep breath. 'Yeah, not feeling much of a man.'

Maureen nodded, slowly, deliberately, maintaining the eye contact as she did so.

Gerry looked away and continued speaking, after taking a deep breath and sighing. He didn't want to talk about the sexual stuff; rather he stayed with how he felt about how he was reacting to his condition. 'I'd really begun to doubt myself as a man. Feeling so sorry for myself, so useless, so bloody useless. But I know that there is more to me than that. I feel like I kind of regained some self-respect. Talking to the kids, and to Carol, that had a big effect on me, and their reaction as well.' Gerry paused. He knew what he wanted to say but he could feel the emotions rising up inside him. His eyes were beginning to water and there was a huge lump in his throat. He swallowed. 'I felt like I came home.' He closed his eyes, the feelings surged through him and the tears rolled down his cheeks. He had his head in his hands and Maureen watched his shoulders moving up and down, juddering as he sobbed.

'Came home to the family, and to yourself as a man.' Maureen was deeply moved by what Gerry was saying and his openness to his feelings. She realised that here was a really sensitive man. She didn't say so; she didn't want to take anything away from what Gerry was experiencing. She sat and bore witness to his outpouring of emotion.

Gerry took a deep breath. Came home, he thought, yes, I've come home, back to what really matters. He knew that his spine was uncomfortable again, as were his feet, but somehow they were less important. He could live with that, so long as he had his family and he felt part of things with them. They really had listened and had sought to reassure him. He had felt their love. He could feel the emotions close to the surface once again.

> Gerry is connecting with feelings about his role in the family, and his own identity, that had been painfully pushed aside in his psychological reaction to his worsening physical symptoms. Now, however, he is able to acknowledge how important his family is, and his role in the family. He is reconnecting with feelings, and as a result integrating them and likely to feel more whole and present.

'Phew.' Gerry had taken in a deep breath and slowly blew the air back out of his mouth. 'That was intense.'

'Lot of emotion, lot of feelings.'

'Yeah. Good feelings, feelings I want to be in touch with. I know it's upsetting but it's good to feel like that. But it takes it out of you.' Gerry was aware of feeling tired all of a sudden. Another symptom of MS. He yawned; he tried to stifle it but to no avail. 'Sorry.' He blinked a couple of times; his eyes were gritty. He was about to say something when he broke into another, longer yawn which left his eyes watering.

'Really has taken it out of you, hasn't it?'

Gerry nodded. And promptly yawned again. He reached over to the cup of water on the table that Maureen must have put out before the start of the session. It was cool and refreshing. It felt good. He felt good, in spite of the tiredness. 'Getting sensitive in my old age,' he joked, smiling as he said it.

Maureen nodded. 'Yes, something like that, but I was thinking just now that you do seem particularly sensitive.'

> Maureen, while being authentic in expressing something that he had been thinking, has unwittingly directed Gerry away from his focus. He now undertakes an exploration of his sensitivity and therefore moves away from the feelings in relation to his role in the family and his sense of being a man. The counsellor really needs to be attentive to the client. She could have said something like, 'Sensitive to a lot of feelings and emotions', which would have held him in his focus while acknowledging the presence of his sensitivity.

'Always have been. Don't know why. I can get emotional over all kinds of things. But I think I'd shut it down in recent months and I was shut down here as well.' Another yawn. 'Oh dear.' He collected his thoughts. 'Where was I?'

'You were talking about being sensitive.'

'Yes, I mean, a romantic film, or some sad ending, or some touching scene and I've gone. I really do react to things like that. Sometimes I wish I wasn't like that but then I think I'm glad that I am. It isn't easy sometimes. I mean, I do avoid some things. Can't watch horror films, stuff like that. I just don't like the feelings in me. It just, well, I don't see the point.'

'I know what you mean, at least, I feel that way too. You just find them too disturbing . . .'

'... yes, that's the word, disturbing. And anything about children being hurt or abused or anything like that.' Even as he said it Gerry could feel his eyes watering again. 'Anything like that and I can feel myself going, it's happening now, just making that comment.'

Maureen nodded and she was aware of wondering where that was arising from. Was he just sensitive, maybe genetic predisposition, or had some experience in life left him with this heightened level of sensitivity? She didn't know and put the wonder aside. She responded to what Gerry had been saying.

'Yeah, anything affecting children badly, that really gets to you.'

'Leaves me feeling sad, angry, empty and I just want to shut it all out.'

'Mhmm, shut it all out. I guess I'm wondering how you do that.'

> Counsellor's issue, not the client's. She didn't need to say anything other than 'shut it all out'. In effect, Maureen has shut out the opportunity for Gerry to focus on his feelings of sadness, anger and emptiness. Could the supervisee be needing to avoid these feelings? She is unaware of what has happened. This is an example of where taping of sessions and listening to them afterwards, or in supervision, can be so beneficial. Supervision relies on the supervisee realising what needs to be explored. A tape can enable them to pick up on what has gone unnoticed during the session.

Gerry shrugged his shoulders. 'If it's on TV I'll turn the channel over or go out of the room. Go and have a drink usually.'

'Anything in particular?' As soon as she said it Maureen realised that it must have sounded odd. She had been wondering if Gerry was using alcohol to dampen down his feelings. She remembered reading a book that had talked about how alcohol could do that, describing the emotions like a fluid jelly, easily prone to wobbling in some sensitive people, and how they could use alcohol to dampen it all down (Bryant-Jefferies, 2001).

'Usually have a beer, I guess, though sometimes I might have a coffee, but usually a beer or two.'

'Helps to take out the wobble?'

'Yeah, that's a good way of putting it. I do feel wobbly and, yeah, the beer calms me down a bit. Funny that.'

Maureen mentioned the book she'd read and that that was why she had said about it taking out the wobble.

'Well, it makes sense to me. But I've always been like that, you know? Even as a child, I couldn't watch some TV programmes. And I still find myself getting upset. I keep away from some films. And I'm not too good with blood either, those programmes showing operations on TV, all in gory detail. Geez, I can't cope with that. When the knife comes out I'm off out – out the door to get some air!'

As Gerry finished speaking Maureen felt a change in the atmosphere. Gerry suddenly looked serious. He had felt quite light in his mood just now, but that had suddenly changed. She wasn't sure why. What had he said? Blood, the knife, operations. Oh, yes, his condition, the possibility of surgery in the future.

Maybe that was what had come to mind. She didn't voice this, rather she enquired what had happened.

Gerry confirmed what she had been thinking. 'Kind of just suddenly had this, well, sort of premonition I guess, you know, I mean, well, I don't know, I may have to have operations in the future. I don't know that I could cope with that.'

'Hard to see yourself coping with major operations, and what we were just talking about brought it to mind.'

Gerry nodded. He took a deep breath. 'But I can't think like that. I've got to get on with today, with what I have, appreciate it, and not spend so much time dwelling on the future, on all the "what ifs" that can so easily take over.'

'Mhmm, need to live for the present and appreciate it . . .'

'That's right. Got to make the best of things.'

Maureen was struck by Gerry's positive tone and how he had managed to switch out of his momentary, well, it had felt like, gloom. 'You seemed to be able to pull yourself out of your gloom just then, and regain a positive sense once more. I'm just struck by that. It seems like a quick change.'

Gerry hadn't thought about it, he had just done it. Yes, she was right. 'Mmm, yes, I did, didn't I? Guess something else has changed. Funny that. There seems to be a lot of change at the moment. Maybe I'm coming to terms with things a little. I don't know. It's still difficult. Still not sleeping well, feeling tired a lot of the time, but I don't want it to get me down, you know? I mean, I really want to face up to things and, well, not give up. I think I'd begun to give up, until I talked at home.' He could feel the tears forming once more in his eyes. 'They were so good, so supportive. I even said to them that it may be that one day daddy will be in a wheelchair. Quick as a flash, do you know what Amy said?'

'No.'

'I'll push you.'

Maureen smiled, aware of feeling lost for words. She lifted her arms and opened her hands as she replied, 'I don't know what to say. Sounds like Amy said it all.'

Maureen is utterly authentic in her response. The recounting of Amy's reaction will have brought feelings and thoughts into Gerry's awareness. He knows what he is feeling and he will choose whether he wishes to convey them to Maureen. Maureen leaves him with what is present for him.

Gerry shook his head, and responded. 'There isn't anything to say. It was so spontaneous, so beautiful, so utterly, utterly genuine. It was like, "OK, we'll sort it out, don't worry", you know? Kids.' He forced a smile and there were tears in his eyes.

Maureen nodded. 'Yes, they can be so matter of fact about things, and so responsive sometimes.'

Gerry shook his head again, briefly closing his eyes. 'In that moment, something happened for me.' He stopped and shook his head again, smiling. 'And Darius, well, typical boy I guess. He reacted quite differently. "You gonna have one of those powered chairs? I'll want a go in it.'' Can you believe it? He loves watching the Grand Prix on TV. I'm sure if he had his way he'd want a red wheelchair with a Ferrari engine in it!'

Maureen smiled, and was aware of feeling deeply touched by the way Gerry was joking about something that in that earlier session he had found it so difficult to talk about, so much fear. 'Nice one. You'll be done for speeding as well!'

'Yeah.' Gerry could smile about it but he was also aware that beneath it the fear remained strong. He could at least make light of it, but he knew that it wasn't something he wanted to really think about much. He was determined to avoid it if he could, and if not, then put it off until he really had to accept it.

'I know we have joked about it, Gerry, but I am aware that maybe that's on the surface. I haven't forgotten the feelings you voiced before about it. Just wanted you to know that.'

Gerry nodded and thanked her. 'I appreciate that. It's partly my way of kind of putting a positive, jokey spin on it, and it was funny at the time, and still is, but it doesn't really take away the thought of what it will be like if it comes to that.'

'No, temporary respite in humour, but the fear, the worry, the not knowing what it will be like in the future remains.'

'And I have to learn to live with that. Can't make it go away. I have to get on and live for the day, as best I can. Enjoy what I can.'

'That sounds very affirming, Gerry.'

Gerry shrugged his shoulders. 'I don't really have a choice, do I? So, I'm starting by taking Darius swimming on Saturday. I think it'll do me good. And it'll be good to do something together – bit of father–son bonding, don't you know!'

'Yes, it's important to you, isn't it, sharing something like that with Darius? What you were saying earlier, you really do want to feel, be, experience being a father to him and not let your condition get in the way of that.'

'No, I don't want it to get in the way. I think he understands, and, well, I'm sure we'll work something out.'

'You sound quite upbeat and positive about it.'

Gerry nodded. 'I am. I feel like the fog has lifted, I feel clearer and, yeah, I'm in a different place.' He stopped, aware that what he was saying was true but also aware that he still struggled to really accept the situation. He still wanted to know why he had this bloody disease, attacking his central nervous system – at least, he was sure that was what it was, giving him so much pain and messing up his life. But he wasn't going to get into that now. The counselling session was leaving him feeling positive and he felt he wanted to leave in that frame of mind. He glanced at the clock: about ten minutes left. He wasn't sure what else he wanted to say. In fact, he really wanted to leave. He had to pick his daughter up from a piano lesson and although he had allowed enough time, assuming the session would end on time, he knew he'd feel a little more comfortable with a few minutes to spare.

'Do you mind if I head off? I really feel that I want to take my positive feelings with me, and I have to pick up my daughter. I know I have time if I stay to the end but it would make it easier.'

Maureen nodded, aware that she wanted to accept Gerry's wish to make a decision that would leave him feeling positive and therefore presumably more satisfied in himself. The session certainly seemed to have been quite full in many ways, and she wasn't going to insist he stayed. Gerry wanted to exercise his autonomy; he had a need to be somewhere and wanted to be sure of getting there on time for his daughter, and he wanted to maintain what he was currently feeling in himself.

They confirmed the time for the following week's appointment and Gerry headed off. He was pleased with how he felt. The counselling had really begun to make a difference. He was being more open with his family and getting back into being a part of things again. He simply hadn't realised how much he had drifted away from them and cut himself off. He realised that this was his way of coping, but he hadn't really coped. It had actually made things worse. It had left him feeling more isolated. He hoped it didn't happen again.

Maureen had written her notes for the session and was thinking about the changes that she had seen in Gerry. There had been a definite shift. He was certainly more relaxed, although, as he had said, the fears about the future remained. They were unlikely to go away; it was more a question of whether he could lead a fulfilling and satisfying life in spite of them. Well, she thought, he's making a start. His family is clearly going to be an important factor in his coping. She knew that there would still be difficult periods, that was how it was. But so long as he used the six sessions that they had to his benefit, that was the main thing. She'd keep listening, keep being there for him.

Halfway through the counselling, she thought, and he has moved more than she had anticipated. She hoped he would build on that, but she also knew she needed to not try to make anything happen, just keep offering the therapeutic qualities: maintain her authenticity, ensure that her empathy was accurate and feel warmth for him. She felt she had been different in that last session as well. She wasn't sure whether it had come across in what she had said, but the last supervision session had made a difference. Although Gerry hadn't talked about his physical pain, she did feel that had he done she could have achieved and communicated an empathic appreciation of what he had communicated.

Anyway, the session was over and she was aware of looking forward to the next session, to finding out how he had got on with his son (assuming he chose to talk about it). Yes, she admired and respected Gerry as he faced up to his progressive disability. No one could say anything to make it better. She had to listen, be a companion, remain a consistent presence for him as he explored himself and his reactions, and talked through his choices and options.

Points for discussion

- Evaluate the style and effectiveness of Donna as a supervisor. What was particularly helpful about Donna's responses to Maureen, and was there anything that seemed inappropriate or unhelpful?

- Discuss the issue of empathising with pain. What do you feel about the notion that it might be different when it is physical rather than emotional or mental?
- Reflect on the nature and quality of Maureen's responses to Gerry. What responses seemed most therapeutically helpful, and why?
- Is Gerry moving towards greater congruence and authenticity within himself and, if so, what is indicative of this?
- Gerry has left early partly to preserve his positive feelings. Is this acceptable?
- Write notes for the supervision session and the counselling session.

CHAPTER 3

Counselling session 4: empathising with pain and realising movement

Gerry was feeling stiff and painful. When he heard his name called he got to his feet. He felt an intense burning pain in his lower back, which ran down his legs leaving his feet tingling as he stood up, felt like someone was running a stream of red hot fire down his legs, in his veins, or somewhere deep within. He gritted his teeth and walked, a little unsteadily, towards the counselling room.

Maureen noticed his difficulty walking. 'Bad day?'

Gerry nodded and sat down, breathing out heavily as he did so. 'Yeah, not so good. Having to work from home. Fortunately they're good about it at work. I've talked it through with my manager and they want to try and be as accommodating as they can for me. Guess they know they've invested a lot in me over the years, I'm still a resource for them.'

'You clearly have a lot to offer.'

'Yes, well, I know the business. I've got good links with our customers and I've got a reputation for getting things done. I'm in the process of focusing some restructuring within the organisation, trying to improve efficiency. Means a lot of juggling of costs at the moment, trying to see where we can make savings without impacting on service. It's coming along. I've been going through the figures today. I'll be presenting my conclusions next week. Meeting with some of the other senior managers. We've all had to do this work for our different sections.'

'So, a lot of figure work and your presentation is next week. You sound confident.'

'I am. Like I say, I know the business, it's more a case of it taking time, getting the details right. I have a good idea what needs to be done. Anyway. That's work.'

'Mhmm. Sounds like you want to talk about something else?' Maureen picked up from the way Gerry was speaking that he didn't want to carry on about work.

'No. Well, I guess I'm feeling sorry for myself again. Not as bad as I was, but not good. I'm trying not to cut myself off again from the family, really trying, but being in pain, well, it's just . . . I can't really explain it, but it's sort of personal, so close, so much part of me, it holds my attention, always there. Dominating everything. It's hard to see, feel, think beyond it sometimes, you know?'

Maureen nodded. 'It kind of dominates, gets in the way of other experiences?' Maureen responded with a questioning tone, wanting to clarify that she was getting a sense of what Gerry was trying to communicate to her.

'Gets in the way of everything. Makes it hard to concentrate on other things. I'm taking some kind of painkillers. It does give some relief, but then it comes back. It's a little easier than at the start of the week, but that was my fault.'

'Your fault?'

'Overdid it in the swimming pool. At least, I think that's what it was. No, I'm sure it was.'

'Did too much?'

'Felt good, the pool was quite pleasant actually, not many people about, and I suppose I was in the best part of an hour. I didn't just swim, I also just moved around. It felt easier at the time. But later, my God. Shooting, stabbing, burning sensation. I could hardly move; when I did it seemed to trigger it off. I was really concerned that I'd done some permanent damage. And my headache flared up again as well. Didn't sleep that night and had to take it really easy on Sunday, just to try and get myself a little more together for Monday. It eased a little, but it wasn't good. And I was so tired. No energy at all.' He breathed out heavily and shook his head. 'Never felt pain like that before. Everything was an effort, you know?' He took a deep breath and sighed. Then yawned; he was feeling tired again now. 'Sorry, still tired. Gets to me, this tiredness. But I do still want to go to the pool; I'm sure I just need to be a little gentler and not spend so much time in it, or maybe just float around more. I don't know. I want to ask the neurologist about it. Darius wants to go again this week and I've said OK, but I'll take it very carefully.'

Maureen listened to Gerry and his graphic description of the pain really impacted on her. It sounded awful. She couldn't begin to imagine what it must have felt like, though she heard clearly Gerry's description.

'I have no concept of the pain you must have been experiencing, or the amount of tiredness you are having to cope with, Gerry. I am so aware of just how personal it is in terms of how you experience it. I can appreciate your feeling you need to kind of shut others out, that it overwhelms you and dominates everything. It does sound like you overdid it, as you say, and I really want to honour your determination to give it another go. That takes courage.'

Maureen was being genuine in what she said. She wanted to be authentic, to let Gerry know that she was hearing what he was saying but how difficult it was to really appreciate the degree of pain he was experiencing.

'Don't know about courage. Maybe foolishness, I don't know, but I have to try. Darius enjoyed himself so much. I just need to learn my limitations – and hope that it won't flare up again in the same way.'

Maureen nodded. 'OK, I appreciate that it doesn't feel like courage to you, but from where I'm sitting it does to me. Either way, Darius is going to appreciate it and, yes, I can appreciate that you don't want it to flare up again. But no doubt it will from time to time. That's the nature of it.' She knew from things she had read recently about multiple sclerosis – she'd got a book on it and had looked up some stuff on the Web. It did flare up for people, and then could settle back down. Sometimes it was clear what had set it off – diet, changes in the weather, overdoing it, lying awkwardly. Sometimes, it seemed to just flare up sponta- neously. The burning, shooting pain that Gerry referred to was what many suf- ferers reported. But she didn't want to start making comparisons. She wanted to hear Gerry, seek to empathically understand what he was experiencing as best she could, and communicate that understanding back to him.

'I just feel like I'm hanging in there, doing what I have to do.'

'Mhmm.'

Gerry continued. 'Just got to find some kind of inner strength I guess to keep on keeping on. But sometimes, and the last few days especially, it's been hard to hold on to that attitude.'

'Feels hard to feel motivated to keep on keeping on when there is so much pain, yeah?'

Gerry nodded. Yes, he thought, some days he just wanted to get out of his body, leave it behind. But he didn't want to die; that wasn't an option. He just felt like he wanted some relief and he knew he got it a little, but this week had been tough.

They sat in silence. Maureen did not feel an urgency to say anything herself. She had sought to let Gerry know that she had heard his last comment, and she waited for him to resume in his own time.

A great deal can be communicated in silences. The person-centred counsel- lor seeks to maintain openness to their own experiencing and attentiveness to their client. They will be sensitive to the tone of the silence and what, if anything, may be being communicated through the presence of the silence. Yet this is undertaken without getting lost in endless speculation which simply detracts from being present for the client.

'Pain's a strange thing. I know I've already said this, but it really is so personal, like no one else can really understand what it is like.' Gerry had spent the silence being so aware of the pain he was currently experiencing. He had been thinking of how we all talk about pain, and use the word 'pain', but we never know exactly how another person experiences it.

'Like it's yours and no one else can really experience what it's like for you.'

'When I spoke to my manager, I mean, he was good, but he couldn't really under- stand what I was saying. I kind of felt that he'd be more sort of, I don't know, able to appreciate or understand more if I had a wound, you know, something he could see, some visible, physical damage.'

'Mhmm, if your manager could actually see damage to your body you kind of think he'd have reacted differently in some way?'

'Yes, like he'd ... I don't know. Just felt like I was having to convince him, you know, I didn't have any evidence. It's all so damned invisible.'

'Nothing to show, no evidence of the damage that is causing the intense pain.'

'And that's difficult. You know, if I had a broken leg then people could see it and know that, yes, there's something wrong there. But with this, what do I have to prove I'm in pain?'

'You feel you need to prove you're in pain?'

Gerry nodded. 'At times, yes. I mean, I know what I'm experiencing, but I can't sort of show it to people. They'll nod and say they understand, which is crap because how can they possibly understand if they haven't experienced it?' He shook his head. 'People don't understand. I guess I'm beginning to get a sense of what it's like to not be normal, well, not like other people. I just have this sense that people think I'm skiving, I mean, they're sympathetic, but ...' He sighed. 'Maybe I'm oversensitive, but I don't think I am.'

Maureen noted the increased volume in Gerry's voice. It clearly angered him, or frustrated him, or maybe both.

'Yes, how can they, anyone possibly understand if they haven't felt what you are experiencing, first hand, so to speak.' Maureen raised the tone of her own voice, seeking to match Gerry, offering him the opportunity to maybe escalate his feelings a little more, engage with them and release them.

'It's frustrating. And you know, and this is so bloody crazy, I end up feeling guilty, like maybe people think there's nothing wrong with me.'

'Feeling guilty because you haven't any visible evidence and you think they think there's nothing wrong with you.'

'And another thing.' Gerry's voice had gone up another notch in volume and he had clenched his right fist. 'And another thing, if someone says to me, "Yes, I know, I get a bit of back pain too" one more time, bloody hell, I feel like I want to punch their fucking lights out.'

Maureen's response did not need agreeing with; Gerry was already moving into a stronger set of feelings. He may not even have heard her.

'Yeah.' Maureen felt her own focus sharpen as she spoke, seeking to catch the intensity of the moment. She decided to repeat back the phrase that Gerry was finding so annoying. 'I know, I get a bit of back pain too. Really helpful, yeah?'

Gerry was shaking his head. He could feel himself tense and his teeth were clenched tight. Bloody idiots, he was thinking. 'They've no idea what it's like. No fucking idea at all. I walk more slowly and more carefully and people get frustrated, I can feel them behind me trying to get past, sometimes they barge into me. Bastards. They have no fucking idea. Do they think I want to be like this? They look at me. You know, I heard someone the other day walk past, look across at me and say to his friend, bloody drunks, should clear 'em off the streets. Bastard. What'll it be like in a wheelchair? Will it be any better? Part of me thinks maybe, but people are so bloody self-centred I wonder.' He was shaking his head again.

'Adds to the hurt, the frustration, the anger. Thoughtless bastards, yeah?'

'Yeah, and I know not everyone's like that. Hell, you seem to understand. And people do sometimes look sympathetically, but not often. Seems like when you're not normal you're in the way. You don't fit. What the fuck have I got to look forward to, hey?' Gerry was shaking his head again. 'But I'm not going to let other people's reactions stop me getting on with my life. But it's so frustrating. What can I do? Nothing. I can't prove what I'm experiencing. Sometimes I have to walk really carefully, you know. Do they think I'm doing that for effect?'

'You wonder, yeah?' Maureen tightened her lips and shook her head slightly.

'I guess I've got to put up with people, but I want to tell them what it's really like, you know, give them a bloody good lecture on it. How it feels never knowing from day to day what amount of pain you'll be in. Not being able to do things that you had planned to do. Pain, always there, grinding you down, taking away any enjoyment. It just takes over, just takes over.'

'Yeah, always there, taking over your day . . . and night.'

'Feels like a bloody prison sentence, sentenced to pain for the rest of your life, and being less mobile, and, shit, there's a whole list of problems associated with MS.' Gerry shook his head. 'Someone up there . . . Oh, what's the point in blaming, I don't know why I've got it, maybe the neurologist will have some answers, I don't know. Last week I started to look up stuff on the Internet. I hadn't realised there were so many symptoms associated with MS. And it's so widespread. It seems to affect people my age or a bit younger, at least to begin with. And I guess I've had some of the symptoms for some while, without realising it. The blurred vision, headaches, tingling sensations in my hands and feet. Just got on with it, you know, put it down to just stress and stuff, but clearly it's been around for a while, and is getting worse . . .' He could feel tears welling up in his eyes. 'Bloody unfair world.'

Maureen waited a moment to be sure Gerry wasn't going to add anything else. She decided not to try and summarise all that Gerry had said, which would stop his process, but to stay with what Gerry had finally said, perhaps thereby letting him continue from where he had left off. 'Hmm, bloody unfair world.'

Gerry knows what he has said, and that Maureen has been listening very attentively. He has developed his thoughts to his final comment, and Maureen responds to the place that Gerry has reached rather than go back over the whole journey. This allows Gerry to know Maureen is attentive but allows him to move on from the point that he has reached with the minimum of delay.

Gerry sat thinking about it. Why were there diseases like this, the symptoms he was at risk of suffering from, well, he couldn't really come to terms with that. Loving God, huh. Didn't feel like that to him. 'I mean, if my kids got it – Christ, I hadn't thought of that. You don't think they may get it, I mean, oh God, it must be genetic.' Gerry looked horrified. Somehow he hadn't really thought about that until now. He wasn't sure why, it suddenly seemed so obvious, but he hadn't. So caught up in his own thoughts about himself, he guessed. 'I need to know, Maureen, oh God, I couldn't ... oh God, no, not that.' He was suddenly aware of a lot of anxiety and his stomach suddenly felt very queasy.

'That thought is ...' Maureen shook her head, struggling to find the right words. 'It's something that ...'

Gerry finished the sentence for her. 'I couldn't face that. But I didn't know. How could I have known. But, no, not that, I'd willingly bear the pain if it would stop it happening to them.' He knew in that moment that he would do that. He was aware of a pressure in his chest, in his heart. Something had shifted. He felt different again. 'I have to check that out with the consultant, see if there are any tests.'

'You'd want them to know?' Maureen knew that she hadn't empathised, but she suddenly felt protective of his children. Would they want to know? She understood Gerry wanting to know, but would they want to know? The whole issue of testing so that people knew was fraught with issues, particularly once it was in the doctor's notes, and could be requested by insurance companies, employers, etc. People live their lives as if they aren't going to be struck down with a particular disease – to carry the thought that you are likely to contract or develop something? And were there tests anyway before symptoms developed? She knew that they tested for lesions in the central nervous system, but ... The truth was, she didn't know. She brought her focus back to Gerry.

Gerry was responding. 'I-I, er, I don't know. I'd want to know.'

'You'd want to know?'

Gerry thought about it. The initial rush of emotion was subsiding. Would he want to know? He'd want to know that they hadn't got it. But what if they had? 'I guess I'd want to know if they were likely to be OK. I guess I'd feel relieved by that, but if they had it or were highly likely to develop it, particularly at an early age ... I don't know. I don't know.' He sighed before continuing. 'I'm being selfish here, aren't I? Thinking of me, my needs. It's no good. But I need to talk about that to the consultant. I think I need a list of my questions.'

'That sounds like a good idea, be sure you raise the issues that you want answers to.'

Gerry nodded and breathed deeply. 'Yes, but that was, well is, a horrible thought. I don't know why I hadn't thought of it before, it's so obvious. I was just so wrapped up in myself, in feeling angry, sorry for myself.' Gerry somehow felt that he needed to have had this conversation with Maureen; it was helping him to adjust his perspective. So many things going on for him, so much to think about, adjust to, make sense of. 'There's just so much going on for me at the moment.' He had tightened his lips again and was looking down at the floor.

Maureen noted the urge to say something to try and make it better and stepped aside from it. That wasn't her role, but being congruent was. 'You know, I'm feeling that I wish I could somehow make it all better, but I know I can't. But the feeling's there. Just wanted you to know that. Stupid thing to say, perhaps.'

Gerry looked up. He swallowed. His eyes were watering again. Oh God, that had sounded good, so genuine, so touching, so caring. 'Thanks.' He swallowed again and closed his eyes. 'I really believe you, and I know you can't do anything except listen. But believe me, it's not only important to be listened to, but more than that, to feel heard, really heard. Remember that telephone ad, "It's good to talk"?'

Maureen nodded.

'Well, they missed the point, what really matters is feeling heard.'

Maureen nodded again. 'Yes, I think, no, I know you're right on that. It's so important to be heard, to know that someone really has taken on board what you are trying to communicate.'

Maureen has made her genuine feelings visible to Gerry. He is touched by them. He feels listened to, he feels heard, he feels, perhaps, the sense of another reaching out into his world. They are personal moments and, without doubt, effective person-centred therapy is personal. The therapist is not there simply as a therapist, but as a person taking the role of therapist, essentially striving to be themselves in therapeutic relationship with another. Their role is to allow the client to explore their inner world and to integrate feelings, experiences, memories and thoughts accurately into their awareness. The counsellor seeks to bring a presence into the relationship, a certain 'quality of presence' that is characterised by, or which takes its nature from, the qualities of unconditional positive regard, congruence and empathy. Such presence is communicated to the client by the counsellors listening and attending to the client as fully as they are able.

'You've listened to me, Maureen, and I've appreciated it. And I've felt heard. It has made a difference. I know it won't change my condition, but it has helped to talk it through and to, I don't know, I kind of find myself seeing things differently, different angles on it, and it isn't that you're giving them to me, just talking about it seems to help me find different perspectives for myself.' He paused, before continuing. 'I guess I burden you up with all my troubles. What do you do with it?'

'Well, I talk it through with a counselling colleague – we call it supervision – and she helps me make sense of my reactions and helps me process anything that arises which might in some way get in the way of your process, that might stop me listening or might leave me wanting to introduce my stuff into the session. It's your time, your space, and I want you to feel free to explore what becomes present for you, what particular issues are arising for you. I'm here to listen, to help you explore and make sense of it all, to provide, or rather offer the opportunity of creating what I'd call a "therapeutic relationship". That may sound a little woolly, but, well . . .'

Gerry interrupted. 'Not to me. It feels sharp and clear. Don't forget I've experienced it, and I know it has helped even though I don't think I could pin down any one thing that you have said. It just feels somehow good, can't think of a better word, having this time to talk. I appreciate it and I want to say thanks.'

Maureen appreciated what Gerry was saying. 'Thanks.' She took time to be with her experience in response to what Gerry had said. She brought herself back to attending to Gerry. She wondered about what to focus on now, and put the thought aside; that was up to Gerry. But she commented, 'So, where does all this leave you now?'

Gerry sat and thought for a while. Ten minutes or so left. He didn't have to rush off and in fact felt in quite a different place in himself to what he did last week at this time, although he couldn't really define that difference to himself. He'd felt good last week, but was anxious about his daughter. He didn't have that anxiety this week. He wanted to stay. It felt good being here. He wanted to stay with that feeling and, yes, maybe explore it a little.

'Kind of leaves me feeling good, somehow. I sort of feel that I'm accepting it a little more, although in saying that I know there's also part of me that doesn't and is angry. But I guess that's how it is.'

'Maybe thinking in terms of different parts is helpful; part of you is accepting, or more accepting, and another part remains angry.'

'It feels easier to think like that. Otherwise, it just feels a tangle with conflicting feelings and, well, it's confusion. I think coming here has somehow helped me to untangle things, and I'm not sure exactly how, but it's to do with talking. And realising the many facets to it as well. But I think I've realised that I have to get on with my life, albeit modified from what I was expecting, and maybe things won't be as bad as they are just now all of the time. I know things are likely to get worse, but there's still life to be lived, and I want to try and get enjoyment out of being with the children, and I want to share good times with Carol, you know?' Gerry felt sad but also determined to make the best of things. He did feel he'd moved on from feeling sorry for himself all the time, which is where he had got to before the counselling.

We might think of Gerry as having integrated painful feelings that he had been pushing away and not acknowledging with his family. He shut down and only really conveyed feeling sorry for himself. His psychological process for coping with the depth of some of these feelings was to go into depression. They overwhelmed him. Emotionally he shut down. Rather like overloading an electric circuit to the point that the trip blows and the system cuts out, Gerry overloaded emotionally and this led to an emotional shutdown, with a preoccupation with what was present in himself because he could no longer cope with taking much in coming from the outside. The counselling has enabled him to slowly begin to switch on some of his emotional circuitry, slowly, gradually, bringing his feelings into awareness and into the therapeutic relationship. Now he is coming to terms with the diagnosis and the implications. It is not that the fear, sadness or anger has gone away – these are all appropriate human reactions to what has occurred – but now they are becoming more manageable as he adapts to and integrates their presence into his functioning sense of self.

Maureen wanted to acknowledge his movement; it seemed so important to Gerry that he could recognise this in himself. 'Yes, I see a shift as well, and I appreciate how important it is for you, and how difficult it must be trying to hold and affirm a positive outlook. You want to enjoy being with your family, do things together and, yes, the future is uncertain, but there is a present to be lived.'

'I was wanting sympathy from everyone before, you know, that's just struck me as you were speaking. That's a big part of the change. That isn't so dominant for some reason, still there, I do want ... no, I don't think it's sympathy, more an appreciation of the fact that there are going to be days when I won't be able to do what I might have wanted to do. I just want people to be able to accept that, but not make a big deal out of it either. That's what I've been doing, isn't it?'

'Making a big deal of it?'

'Yes, and as I say that I want to also say that it is a big deal, and I have a right to see it that way as well.'

'Mhmm, sure, you have a right to make a big deal of it if you want to, yes?' Maureen spoke with an attitude of belligerent assertiveness.

Gerry nodded. 'And no.' He shook his head. 'Oh, I don't know. I can get caught up in words sometimes, I think, and end up confused. I think what I am trying to say is that OK, there will be times, there are times, when I'm going to feel sorry for myself and I want to be left to do that, but at the same time I don't want to burden others with it – well, my family basically. I think that's where I'm at with it.'

'Sounds clear to me, you want to feel able to feel sorry for yourself, but you don't want to burden your family with your feelings?'

Gerry nodded again, in a slow and thoughtful way. 'Hmm. Yes. And maybe it'll go into remission for a while. It does happen. One of the websites described different types of MS, and, well, I've got to be optimistic. I mean, it's not all bad, I have good periods, maybe it won't be as bad as I fear. It's just ...' He paused. 'It's just so easy to be anxious about it. I guess, you know, typical man, don't go to the doctor for years about symptoms, and then when you do, you start worrying about it, and trying to deny it's happening, but you can't. Anyway, I'm seeing the doctor at the end of the week, I want to talk to him again about the symptoms. He gave me some information about MS some while back, printed it off from his computer. I've managed to lose it. Well, I don't think I really wanted to read it. I guess I put it somewhere, but I don't know where. I want another copy and this time, well, I feel ready to really read up on it and start to get to grips with it. And I guess I want to get a basic understanding before I see the consultant in, what, two weeks now.'

'So that's another shift. Before you didn't want to know, now you're wanting information.' Maureen had glanced at the clock. 'Time's nearly up, and that seems to be a rather positive note on which to end the session. However, is there anything else you wanted to say?'

Gerry shook his head. 'No. Thanks again. I'll see you next week. Same time?'

'Yes.'

'OK, I'll see you then. Bye.'

'Bye. Take care.'

'Yes, will do, certainly will on Saturday when I go to the pool again with Darius. I'm gonna take that really carefully!'

'Yes, I feel sure that you will.'

Counselling session 5: what is multiple sclerosis?; the client experiences a remission

'Well, the swimming went well, took it very carefully. Got a bit of a reaction but in fact it feels like things have settled down somewhat. I'm feeling more mobile again, less of the shooting pains and the headache has eased.'

'Mhmm. That must be a relief.'

'Yes. I mean, I know it may not last, well, probably won't, but it's good to have a bit of respite from it. Just mustn't forget and overdo it in case it flares up again.'

'Easy to do, I guess, in a moment of forgetfulness.'

'Yes. I have to be careful on that. Anyway, I had a chat with the GP and he's printed out the information sheet. I've been going through it. Have you seen it?'

'No, I haven't, and I really ought to have a copy.' Maureen had meant to get one for herself but she hadn't, and she wasn't sure what that was about. Anyway, she would make it her first action after the session. Someone was sure to know how to do it, or she'd ask one of the doctors.

'I'm sure I did read through it before but I don't think I'd taken it in. Now I feel I've got an understanding of it. It's amazing what they say happens.'

'Mhmm.'

'It seems there is still some uncertainty as to the cause, but it's to do with the auto-immune system. There might be a viral factor involved, but either way the body attacks itself and lesions are created in the central nervous system. Something called myelin is attacked, which affects how information gets transmitted along the central nervous system. It gets inflamed and can lead to scarring, and that's what the sclerosis is, the scarring. The GP again said how difficult it can be to diagnose and that the neurologist would run tests, and that it might take a while to be absolutely sure. But he agreed I was describing symptoms that were very typical of the condition.'

'So, you have a much clearer idea of what it is.'

'Yes. And I asked about whether it was genetic and, well, it is but it's by no means definite that children get it as well, though the risk is increased. He kind of reassured me on that. But it doesn't seem that there are tests, it's difficult to diagnose.'

'Hmm, that had been really troubling you.'

'Yes, but he has reassured me I think, the risk is still low even though it is higher than it would be for anyone else. Apparently it affects women more than men.'

'Mhmm.'

'And there are no absolutely conclusive tests for it, but a range of tests which, together with the symptoms, go together to lead to a diagnosis. They apparently can do magnetic resonance imaging [MRI] in some way that I didn't fully understand, but it means they can see whether any of the lesions are sort of active or something, and helps them rule out other possible causes. But they also need to do different neurophysiological tests as well, to check the way neurological messages are transmitted. Probably have me strapped to some electrical gadget for that. They can test the speed of signals reaching the visual cortex and that can indicate whether there is damage.'

'Sounds pretty technical stuff.'

'It is. So I can expect to be wired up and maybe scanned. They can also take fluid from your spine which can indicate chemical changes, though they may not do this because the MRI scan can give them the information they need. I hope it doesn't come to that, sounded painful.'

'Yeah, doesn't sound too pleasant.'

'So that's where I'm at with it. And since then, well, a bit tingly on Sunday after the swimming trip, but otherwise things feel like they have settled down a bit. Apparently these sort of flare-ups can occur quite frequently, but people experience MS in different ways. For some people it is simply progressive, for others, it can be sort of in cycles, and it seems that the cycles themselves can become progressively worse, but again, not everyone, so it is uncertain.'

'Yes, you must be hoping that you get long periods of, what, a kind of remission, between these cycles.'

'I hope so. But I'm relieved that the symptoms have worn off a little and, well, that things are a little easier. My sleeping has improved. In fact, I seem to be catching up, going to bed quite early and sleeping through.'

Maureen had a question. 'So how many people on average suffer with it?'

Gerry is clearly wanting to share his knowledge and his understanding of the disease. Maureen gets caught up in information mode, hence her question. However, it conveys an interest in what Gerry is saying. He wants to talk this way and in a real sense she has facilitated this. The person-centred counsellor wishes to convey warm acceptance of the client as they are, within their reality, and as they communicate what, at the time, they most want or need to express.

'Now I read that in some other information booklet.' Gerry thought for a moment. 'I think it was around 80 000 or maybe a little more, something like that. Sounds like a lot of people and yet, compared to other diseases, I guess it is relatively small. And yet they don't seem to really fully understand the cause.'

'Yes, it is surprising. You'd think that, by now, someone would have. But as you say, maybe the consultant will have more up-to-date information, or at least be able to tell you a little more.'

'Yeah, I'll have to wait and see.' He lapsed into silence. He wasn't sure what to say now. Felt pleased with himself that he had remembered so much about it. He really wanted to understand what it was he was up against now. Felt like sort of trying to get to know the enemy. He voiced his thoughts. 'I want to know what I'm fighting, you know, what the enemy's like, what I can do to sort of fight it off, so to speak.'

'Must feel like a battle, a battle that's just beginning.'

Gerry took a deep breath. 'Yes.' Yes, he thought, it is just beginning and it's likely to be lengthy unless he was one of the lucky ones and it turned out to be a mild form. He hoped that was the case but somehow he didn't think so. It was the stabbing pain he had been experiencing that left him doubting that it would be mild in the longer term. And, of course, the bouts of tiredness that could really drag his mood down. But he could only wait and see.

Maureen waited for Gerry to continue. It had felt quite conversational through most of the session so far. Gerry obviously had felt he wanted to talk about what he had learned about his condition, and Maureen respected that.

Clients don't always want to talk about what some might term 'issues'. Sometimes it is a kind of reporting back on the week, or a sharing of some new insight that they are enthusiastic about. Gerry is feeling good. His pain and stiffness has eased. He's much closer now to seeing the consultant. He's likely to be in a different frame of mind.

'So, all in all, things feel a lot easier. We've decided to book a holiday. It's a bit of a risk, obviously things could become problematic again for me, but, well, we'd do nothing if we just let ourselves worry about that. We haven't decided where to go yet, but we'll sort that out.'

Maureen found herself thinking about how Gerry was now looking ahead in a positive manner. 'The thought struck me just then how you are now looking ahead. So much changes when the pain is reduced, or maybe it's more than that . . .'

'It is more than that, but you're right, feeling the pain and tiredness reduce does leave me feeling more hopeful. And seeing the consultant soon, that's a factor too. When I was first told how long a wait it would be, it seemed like an eternity. All I knew was that I had reached a point where I had to admit to myself that something was wrong, and I wanted it dealt with, straight away. It's been a long wait, at times it felt interminable. But now I kind of feel things are happening, positive things, and I want to make the most of it, and of feeling the way I do.'

'Mhmm, make the most of the mood you're in. That feels really important hearing you say that.'

Gerry nodded. 'I have to. I have to, you know?'

'Yes. You have to make the most of it.'

Gerry was all too aware that he had no idea what time frame he was in insofar as how long he would feel the way he did at the moment. But he was going to make the most of it. Do things at weekends. Maybe get some stuff done around the house as well, though he didn't feel he wanted to make that his number one priority.

The counselling session continued with Gerry talking about the kind of things he hoped to do, and how he really wanted to make it up to his family for how he had been over recent months. He was genuinely sad about how it had been, and talked of his feelings of guilt. Maureen listened and offered her empathic appreciation of not only what it had been like, but how it was feeling for him now.

'I don't want to get like that again, but I know the likelihood is that I will, if it all gets too much again. I guess it's my way of coping, closing down, turning in on myself, shutting other people out. I guess it's what other people do as well, I don't know.'

'Like it's your style – is that the right word? – the way you look after yourself, closing down and cutting yourself off.' Maureen wasn't sure about style, felt maybe more of a habit or just a way of coping that Gerry had learned and repeated.

Gerry nodded. 'I've talked to Carol again about it, well, we just talk more openly about it more often now, and she said it was really difficult, feeling shut out, unable to do anything. She said she felt helpless and was really worried as to how long it would last. She said she was so relieved when I said I was going to counselling. She'd had counselling herself, many years ago, after her sister died suddenly in a car accident. They were really close, and I know she found it helpful, helped her come through it. So, yes, she was really pleased.'

'Mhmm. So difficult for her feeling shut out, but really pleased you came to counselling. Must have had a big effect on your relationship.' Now why did I say that, Maureen thought, that's directive, but it's said now. She put it down to her curiosity; Gerry hadn't really said a great deal about his relationship with Carol. But it wasn't appropriate although it had been said now. Still, Gerry has the choice whether to respond or not. But she knew it hadn't been a very person-centred response although Gerry had been talking a bit more about Carol.

'Things have improved a lot. We'd got to a real kind of silent stand-off at times. She couldn't get close, and I wouldn't let her get close. But I am concerned it'll happen again, and I've tried to explain to her.'

'Explain?'

Maureen has gone with the issue of explaining, which is where Gerry ended his comments, rather than trying to convey her empathic understanding of all that he has said. He is thereby allowed to develop this theme.

'Why I do it. I'm protecting myself. I've always been a bit like that. I'd kind of withdraw if I felt threatened or vulnerable. I'd just kind of retreat, clam up, get away from things that I couldn't handle. I was like that at school. I'd kind of keep myself to myself a lot of the time. Never really at the centre of things, always on the edge looking on, keeping my distance.'

'So something stopped you from being at the centre, kept your distance, kept yourself to yourself.' Maureen was wondering where, if that style was already establishing itself at school, it had originated.

'Yes, don't really know why. I wasn't like that at primary school. Went to a small school and I kind of was very much at the centre of things there. Yes, that was different, thinking about it. But later, I seemed to be different somehow.'

'So, at the centre of things in primary school but something changed when you went to secondary school.'

'Yes. It was a big school, I remember that, and I found it hard to adjust. So many kids, and, well, I think looking back it was all a bit overwhelming to me. Took me a long time to adjust, in fact, I'm not sure that I ever did, not really. But at university it was different again. Seemed much more in the social thick of things there. Out drinking and stuff, you know?'

A bell went off in the back of Maureen's head. Alcohol. Gerry had said something about having a few drinks to relax himself after that first session, and how he drank to cope with his sensitivity, particularly towards children. She just sensed there was something there, but she wasn't sure what, and it was a connection she was making anyway, and not something Gerry seemed to be concerned about. But it somehow nagged at her, it felt . . . she wasn't sure, but it was such an instantaneous reaction and connection that came into her head. She decided to trust her reaction and voiced it in the form of a question.

Maureen is trusting her own instincts. Voicing what she is thinking is likely to be more therapeutically valid where it emerges from a sense of connection with the client. In this instance, it has the flavour of spontaneity – the experience of 'a bell going off'. She expresses what has become present for her.

'It kind of reminds me how you said about having a few drinks to cope with feeling disturbed, and I guess I'm wondering if it helped you settle into university in some way?'

He hadn't thought of that. He had drunk quite a lot at university, but then everyone did, or seemed to. 'Well, yes, but I wasn't really thinking like that. Just found I could relax and be part of things.' He stopped and thought about it some more. He'd started drinking before university, but it hadn't been so important somehow, but that had changed when he was away from home. 'I guess I did drink to get confidence. I hadn't really mixed much. I mean, my sister was a lot older than me, and her friends never wanted to have much to do with me when they came around. I had friends at school, and we'd get together and do stuff, but I kind of felt awkward sometimes. Don't know why. Maybe I carried that into university. But I think I got over it.' He paused. 'You're right, though, I do drink to feel relaxed sometimes, take the edge off things and probably my drinking did go up in recent months.'

'And it can bring your mood down, and it may have added to that, and heavy drinking can disturb sleep patterns.'

'I hadn't realised it had that effect.'

'Yes, not many people do. But you feel you've got over some of that tendency to be on the edge of things, of keeping yourself to yourself, though it kind of reappeared somewhat in recent months.'

'Yes. And I know I must watch that. I don't want to shut Carol out, or the children, you know? They're important, very important.'

'Really important.'

Gerry nodded and could feel his emotions rising. That sensitivity again. He looked at the clock; time was nearly up. 'OK, so, I think that's all I want to say today. Next week I'm seeing the consultant and then it's our last session, and that feels OK too.'

'Yes, so you may want to think of how you want to use that last session. Maybe review the process here, or maybe think about what needs you may still have and how they can be met, or, well, whatever is with you.'

'Yes. I guess I'll see what the consultant has to say first and then I guess I'll maybe want to explore things depending on what he has said. I don't know.'

'Sure. So, see you in two weeks. I hope the meeting with the neurologist goes well.'

'Thanks.'

Maureen sat back in the chair after Gerry had left and reflected on how much he had changed. She realised that some of it was reactive to his symptomatology, but she felt that he had moved on a lot since that first session. She felt good about the work that they had done together and she hoped that she was helping to help Gerry find the strength and the perspective on his health problem that would enable him to cope with it. She knew six sessions of counselling wasn't long, but she also knew from experience that it could still make a huge difference for people. And of course, she knew he could always refer back if he felt he needed to address something, or if things got worse and he was struggling again. She wrote up her notes and started to collect her things together ready to head home.

Points for discussion

- What aspects of the last two sessions stand out for you in terms of therapeutic significance, and why?
- Did the almost conversational feel to parts of the last session seem appropriate? What role did they have from the perspective of person-centred theory?
- What evidence did you note that a therapeutic alliance had developed between Maureen and Gerry?
- Evaluate Maureen's empathy towards Gerry's pain.
- Was it right for Maureen to raise the alcohol issue in the way that she did? Would you have made a similar comment? Can it be justified in terms of person-centred working?
- Write notes for these two sessions.

CHAPTER 4

Supervision session 2: empathy, alcohol and feelings for Gerry explored

'I want to turn to my work with Gerry, you remember, the client with the possible MS whose mood had lowered and who we talked about last time in terms of my struggle to empathise with his pain?'

'Yes, I remember. You were struggling with how much you could empathise with his experience and, yes, talking about the fact that you were healthy and what impact that had on your empathy, yes?'

'Yes. Well, a lot has happened. It's hard to know exactly where to begin.'

'Mhmm. A lot going on, then?'

Maureen nodded and thought about what to say first.

> She had been thinking about what she wanted to say before the session; she always prepared her thoughts although she knew that supervision could take you in unexpected directions, particularly when your awareness opened up to aspects of the therapeutic relationship and the impact it was having on a counsellor's ability to offer quality empathy, congruence and unconditional positive regard. But she always felt that the preparatory work seemed to make the supervision process more focused and helpful. That was her experience; she was sure that other counsellors worked in different ways that suited them.

'I want to begin by saying that last session was really helpful. It did free me up and I think I was much more sensitive and responsive as a result, particularly the session where Gerry talked about his pain, what it was like. It sounded really debilitating.'

'Good, I'm glad it was useful. So, his pain, debilitating, but you found yourself more freed up to listen and respond empathically?'

'I think so. He talked about how he hadn't really talked much to his family, kind of shut them out. Last session, he went on to reflect on how this pattern seemed to have run from childhood, particularly during his time at secondary school. And then he talked about – well, I introduced it – about his use of alcohol at university to damp down discomforting feelings.'

'You say you introduced it. I'm wondering what that was about.' Donna wasn't sure how that was going to fit with Maureen's non-directive, person-centred practice. She wanted to check it out to ensure that Maureen's issues were not clouding the quality of her empathy.

'Well, he'd talked in a previous session – since I last saw you – about his sensitivity. He struggles watching certain programmes on TV, particularly, now what did he say, programmes where there were operations with blood and stuff. He said he would sometimes walk out of the room and go and have a drink to settle himself down. Not always alcohol, but certainly it figured as a feature of his coping strategy.'

'And how did that develop?'

'Well, we didn't really get into that very much. I can't recall now how the session developed; I kind of noted it but felt that he was simply telling me what he was doing and I sought to listen and let him know that I was hearing him, and that I had an appreciation of what he was experiencing. Oh yes, that leads me on to something else I wanted to explore. But I'll come back to that. Anyway, he then mentioned in a later session about his difficulty at secondary school, how he had kept himself to himself, but how at university he was more able to be at the centre of things, and he mentioned drinking as part of the culture, and I asked him about it. I was wondering whether he had been using it then as a way of coping with his sensitivity, in the context of boosting his sort of social and self-confidence. Anyway, he thought that maybe he did. So I guess I didn't introduce it, but rather I kind of flagged it up – probably directed him towards it. But I was, well, I guess, no, I know, my concern was and is whether he's at risk of it getting out of control, you know? If he's using it to cope in some area of his life, how much it might become a feature of his coping with the MS, particularly if it gets worse which it seems that statistically it is likely to do.'

'That's the ex-alcohol counsellor in you coming out, isn't it?'

'Yes, and I know that, but I don't want to deny my concern, you know? I kind of internalised a lot of awareness around alcohol use during that placement with the community alcohol team and, even though it was for a short time, it made an impression on me. I don't know, I like Gerry, I'd hate to see him wind up with an alcohol problem on top of everything else if it could be avoided. Alcohol affects the central nervous system and, well, if it is MS he's suffering from, it can't be helpful if he drinks heavily and must be likely to add complications.'

'Mhmm. You care about him, you don't want him to risk doing more damage or complicating his health.'

'Yes, and I respect him in many ways. I mean, I only see him as he is with me, but I guess I've really tuned in to the immensity of what he is facing up to. And yes, I want to help, make some difference in the sense of helping him come through this period of his life in a way that helps prepare him for the future.'

'I guess we all want to make a difference; it's whether we are open to the client's process taking them to their difference, or whether we are carrying a sense of the difference that we think the client ought to make or experience and then we try to direct them towards it.'

Donna affirms clearly the principle of person-centred working that requires the counsellor to be open to the client's needs, goals and agendas. The more the counsellor carries in their mind (even if it is not directly voiced) a specific goal for the client there will be a risk that they will subtly seek to direct them towards it. Whether or not the counsellor has a goal for the client is an ongoing person-centred debate. Perhaps that goal, if there is to be one, is for the client to achieve an increasingly authentic experience of themselves. However, maybe a more person-centred goal would be simply that of offering the core conditions in the knowledge that, for the therapist, the creating of a therapeutic relationship *is* the key to constructive personality change.

Maureen thought for a moment. 'I guess for me it's about, well, I felt really good when he talked about how talking to me had encouraged him to talk to his family. I think it was the session after our last supervision. He had decided he needed to level with his family about how he felt about things, but mainly to explain to the children what was happening. And it was so touching. The children responded really positively.' She could feel her eyes watering and a lump in her throat as she continued. 'His daughter said she'd push his wheelchair, and their reaction made a huge impact on Gerry. He seems much more part of the family now, and at the last session he was saying that it felt like the pain was easing, that maybe he was in some kind of remission. Apparently it flares up for people and the experts still don't really know exactly what causes MS, although they have an idea what is happening in the body and it seems to be linked to the auto-immune system. Gerry started to go swimming with his son and overdid it, and that set it off and he had a really bad time with it. It set off a lot of tiredness and that was when he really talked more about the pain. It seems that he is opening up, trusting people with what must be leaving him feeling so vulnerable.'

Donna had been struck by what Maureen had said about Gerry's daughter's reaction. She had noticed Maureen's voice get a little emotional at that point. 'I'm struck by the level of your own emotional sensitivity towards Gerry and his situation. He must feel that you are affected. I think it is so important in person-centred working that we allow how we are affected to be visible. I mean, obviously, we don't spend the whole session going on about how we feel, but it is important.'

'I agree, and I'm sure that it is why I probably held him on the alcohol issue a bit, I could just see how it might get out of control. But I didn't sort of say anything really directive like, "Don't drink like that", you know? And I wonder if I'll be tempted to say something in the last session we are having, you know, something like, "And watch the booze doesn't become too much of a coping mechanism''. But even as I say that now, it doesn't feel right. I mean it does, but it doesn't. Feels like I'm imposing my frame of reference on him, but then I also want to try and help him avoid a possible problem, and I want to be authentic.'

When a person-centred counsellor has knowledge or information that might be of value or helpful to the client, is it acceptable to introduce it? Maureen has knowledge of how patterns of alcohol use can indicate a coping strategy that could become a problem. She wants to be authentic.

If the counsellor holds back on a piece of information, are they clouding their authenticity? Put yourself in the position of the client: would you want your counsellor to be open about information or concerns that they might have, genuinely held concerns?

The person-centred counsellor seeks to offer unconditional positive regard. So long as the counsellor does not convey a value judgement on the client or their choices, thus risking undermining them and introducing a 'condition of worth', it seems reasonable that genuine concerns or known and relevant pieces of information be conveyed.

'I really do appreciate what you are saying here; you think you may be feeling an urge to impose your frame of reference on Gerry, and I guess it's about resolving or rather getting clarity on what are your needs and what are Gerry's.'

Maureen smiled. 'My need is to make a positive difference, and feel that I've said what I want him to hear.' Maureen grimaced. 'What I want him to hear. That's not very person-centred of me.'

'Why do you say that?' Donna hoped Maureen would explore this further. It felt to her like an issue of appropriate congruence but she wanted to let Maureen work towards her own conclusion on it.

'Well, it's not so much an emphasis on me being transparent. It's got an edge to it.'

'So it's not appropriate for that edge to be made transparent.'

Maureen stopped and thought about that. 'What I said earlier, about saying something like watching that the alcohol doesn't become too much of a coping mechanism, could come out like a kind of verbal pointed finger, if you know what I mean, a kind of ''and another thing'', and I really don't mean it like that.'

'Mhmm, OK, so you don't want to, as it were, point the finger at him through the language you use. So what do you want him to hear?'

The response was very present and immediate, the moment Donna asked the question. 'I want him to know that I care.'

'OK, care about . . . ?'

'About him and his well-being.'

'You really don't want him to make things worse, yes?'

Maureen nodded.

'So how else might you say what you want him to hear? What would be really authentic?'

'I guess my concern that the alcohol may end up as a problem.'

'OK, so how might you say that to Gerry.'

Maureen wasn't sure. It felt kind of awkward trying to find the right words. She felt sure they would emerge out of the experience of being with Gerry. But then maybe this wasn't about finding the words that she would use; maybe it was more about connecting with what was present in her that she wanted to make visible. Maureen pushed aside the idea that she had to find the right way to say it. She simply had to find a way to say it and hear herself, feel herself, connect with what it was.

Maureen started to speak. ' "I also want you to know that I am a little concerned that, well, go easy on the alcohol", no, I'm still telling him what to do, aren't I?'

'Is that how it feels to you?'

Maureen nodded. 'I'm making it all too complicated here, getting myself tangled up in words. I want him to know I care, I'm concerned, and I want to flag up the alcohol use as a potential problem.'

'Mhmm.'

'So I need to acknowledge all that but simply. "I need to say that I'm concerned that you may . . ." No, I've lost it. Am I trying too hard here?'

'Maybe.'

'I think I am. I think I really need to let my words emerge out of the contact we are having in that last session. I know I have something I want to say, that I need to own my concern, acknowledge that it is my stuff in a way, but that it feels important to me.'

Donna felt she could trust Maureen to find her own words in the context of the moment when it arose within the therapeutic relationship. It seemed that Maureen had worked on it in this session, had clarified the issue, and now she should be trusted to act in a professionally personal way with her client.

Sometimes in supervision it is about raising awareness and not coming to a definable solution. What Maureen will say, what will be appropriate, cannot be generated in supervision. It will emerge in the context of the therapeutic relationship. The person-centred counsellor trusts the process that is present both for the client and for themselves, and which overlaps within the therapeutic alliance.

'I want to say that I trust you to find the appropriate words to convey what you need to say if and when the time arises.'

Maureen appreciated that. She felt herself becoming less tense. 'Thanks for that. Yes, I'm sure now that I've spent some time processing this it'll come together. I'm aware of the time and I do want to just explore something else that has come up for me, and I think it is my experience of working with Gerry that has highlighted this for me. It is something about empathic appreciation and empathic understanding. I'm still trying to make sense of it, but it kind of feels important somehow. It's like I'm not sure that I can empathically understand Gerry in terms of his physical pain, but I can appreciate the kind of effect that pain can have. And it kind of left me wondering about empathic understanding, and what it actually is. I know it is about being able to move around within the client's inner world or frame of reference, but I find myself drawn to thinking about it more and more in terms of appreciating that inner world than necessarily understanding it. I may be playing with words, but it somehow feels important, you know how bits of theory sometimes get to you?'

Donna nodded. 'OK, let me see if I'm understanding you.'

'Hold it, you said "understand".'

'Yes, but at the moment I don't know if I do understand you. So I am going to say what I think I understand by what you have just said.'

'OK.'

'So, my understanding is that you are not sure whether you can empathically understand what is present within the client's inner world, but that you can maybe more accurately describe what you experience as an appreciation of what is in their inner world.'

Maureen was aware that what Donna had said sounded really good and yet she wasn't sure it was quite what she had said. 'Ah, so what I'm now thinking then is that I am empathically understanding my client's description of their inner world, not their actual inner world as they experience it.'

'You can't experience a client's inner world; that is theirs. We can maybe, using your word, appreciate what it is composed of. But the understanding is related to what the client is telling us about that inner world. Is that right? I think that's how it seems for me.'

'This is really helpful. I think I've somehow got myself tangled up on what I am trying to empathise with, and maybe there are two sorts of empathy operating: empathic understanding of what the client is communicating, and empathic appreciation of our sense of what the client's inner world is like. And I'm not sure how much the two overlap, but I guess my hope is that they will.'

'Could it be that empathic understanding of what the client says enables us to empathically appreciate the content of their inner world?'

Maureen sat and thought about that. 'It's like there are two things: the reality of the client's inner world, and that is private to them, and there is their communicating of that world, and sometimes maybe that world cannot be described or put into words. I guess it has come up because I know I can understand what Gerry tells me about his experience, but I cannot actually fully understand that experience because it isn't mine.'

'And your struggle with being healthy and pain-free, while he is not, sort of highlighted this struggle to get an understanding of his world?'

'I can't, and it was the word "understanding" that was the problem. But I can appreciate something of that inner world, what it must be like, although I cannot understand it. Oh, I'm struggling with words again. Seems like a theme today.'

'Mhmm, struggling with words, with finding words to convey what you want to say. Let me say something here. I understand that you are struggling with words today, and I appreciate how frustrating that must be. Does that help?'

'Yes, and no, because I think it's the other way around. Maybe you appreciate my struggle with words but you understand my frustration.' Maureen closed her eyes. 'I'm getting lost here, but there is something for me in all of this, but I can't seem to get hold of it.'

Supervision sessions may not always focus on specific clients or a counsellor responding to a particular client. Sometimes theoretical issues develop out of the work with a client, and these can be usefully explored. Here, Maureen is confused over the nature of empathy and her struggle as to whether she can understand a client's inner world, particularly, as in this case, a world that she has no parallel experience of.

'Something slightly out of reach, something . . .' Donna held the silence, allowing herself to be with her wanting Maureen to resolve this tangle over words and their meaning, and what she experienced when she talked about empathy.

'It's about my sense of what the client is telling me about their inner world, and my lack of sense of that inner world. I can enter into what their words tell me, but I can't get into what is behind the words, what is actually the reality being described. Yes, I can empathise with the description, but not the thing described. It's something like that. And I'm trying to find words to convey this. And I'm not sure now which way around it is, but I want to use understanding and appreciation to try and differentiate empathy for the client's description of their inner world, and some kind of empathy for that inner world as it actually is. I'm getting clearer here. It's whether my only way of knowing my client's inner world is through their description, or whether there may be times when, through maybe intuition, I can actually somehow directly appreciate the content of their inner world, and that appreciation is like a sixth sense. It can be right but I could fool myself with a hunch, or draw from my own experience, and then it wouldn't be accurate. That feels OK to me now, but how's it left you?'

'I think that the issue as you now describe it may have been behind the issue as you originally introduced it. It's like, can I directly apprehend my client's world in some way that bypasses what they tell me about it. Can that be trusted? Is it authentic? And, yes, I kind of agree that it is something to do with intuition. I remember reading something about intuition as being utterly reliable when it is genuine intuition. But often it isn't, it's a mixture of hunch and guesswork, and a "feels right" factor, which cannot necessarily be trusted. Anyway, it's been helpful talking like this.' Maureen glanced up at the clock.

Time had passed by. 'Time's nearly up,' Donna commented, noticing Maureen's glance. 'Has all this been helpful? It's certainly got me thinking. Do you feel ready for your final session with Gerry?'

'Yes, I do. I feel – hard to describe – somehow more composed I guess. I'm going to miss him. I feel like we have really made a connection, you know, real person-to-person stuff. Feels good. I'm sure I'll need to process the ending though at our next session.'

'Sure.'

The session drew to a close. Maureen left feeling quite thoughtful. She wasn't yet completely clear on exactly how she saw empathy, but she felt that there were different types, qualities, depths – she wasn't sure what was the right word to use. She knew she would ponder on this more; it was something that fascinated her. And it did feel relevant to Gerry as it had been her struggle to empathise with his pain that had really sowed the seed for her musings. One more session to go. She wanted it to be a helpful ending, a real sense of transition. So often she felt endings were focused solely on the stopping aspect of ending, whereas she had found in her experience, and with her clients, that the ending required an honouring of the new beginning that will surely follow, even if it is only a beginning of a period without the experience of ongoing counselling, though more often than not the client was looking for ways to move on.

Counselling session 6: more about multiple sclerosis and an ending with smiles

Gerry had had a good week. The remission had continued. He was feeling more like he had done months back, before he'd been to the doctor the first time to try to find out what was wrong. He was in a good frame of mind. He had also got on well with the consultant; she had seemed to really appreciate his difficulty and the effect it was having on him. So he was in buoyant mood when he saw Maureen heading into the waiting room. He got up and walked towards her.

'Hi. Nice day out there.'

'Yes, hope it lasts.'

'They reckon it will, for a few days anyway. So it looks good for the weekend at least.'

They had reached the door of the counselling room. The surgery had its own room purposely designed for counselling. This was something Maureen very much appreciated. She had worked out of other rooms in the past, and been so aware of the intrusive nature of the medical environment. She waited for Gerry to sit down, and she sat down herself.

'So, how are things and how do you want to use our time in this last session?'

'I was just thinking about what I was saying just then about the weather. You kind of hope it will last, but you know it will change eventually, but you don't know when. Seems to be a good metaphor for me at the moment.'

'Something about not knowing when there will be change?'

Gerry nodded. 'Yes. I'm actually feeling good, physically well and mentally as well. The pain has gone, just a little bit of uncertainty when I walk sometimes but nothing really significant. I had a long chat with the consultant and she was really helpful. Gave me more information, ran some tests and has arranged an MRI scan. Said she felt it seemed likely that it was MS. Somehow she seemed confident and reassuring. Not that she really did anything, but, I don't know, somehow it felt reassuring to have someone on the case who really seemed like she knew what she was talking about. I mean, that's not to say that the GP doesn't, he does, but she . . . well, I guess it's because she's a specialist. So, yes, Mrs Suliman was her name. It was really helpful.'

'So something about the way she was, her knowledge, left you reassured.'

Gerry nodded. 'I'd waited so long for that appointment and I was actually quite nervous beforehand. I really was wondering if I was going to be disappointed, whether I might just feel I was on a conveyor belt, or whether I'd actually see the consultant rather than a junior, you know?'

Maureen understood exactly what he meant. 'A lot of uncertainty but must have been a relief to know you were talking to the top person.'

'Yes, precisely. And, well, you don't mind me telling you more about it?'

'No, not at all, so long as you are sure it is how you want to use some of the session today.'

'I feel I do need to talk to you about it. Somehow you've been very much part of my kind of, I don't know, well, sort of journey, I suppose, these past few weeks. I kind of feel I want you to know about it and the outcome.'

Maureen was genuinely interested although she would not have asked Gerry had he not been forthcoming. She was genuine in her response. 'I'd really appreciate hearing what you have to say about it, what happened, what suggestions have been made.'

Another example of the counsellor trusting the client to know what their needs are, and offering unconditional acceptance of their need to talk about something important to them. In a sense it helps the client to feel that what they have evaluated as being important has an external worth as well. What is important to them is important to another. It fosters their trusting of their own judgement.

Gerry somehow felt validated in some way, like something important to him was being acknowledged as important to someone else. It encouraged him to continue. 'The tests – wired me up and measured signals reaching my visual cortex – she said the timing was out, that there was something happening to block the signals. She took a long history of my symptoms. She explained a lot of the things I'd read, but somehow I sort of heard it more clearly. I think it was her sensitivity and her confidence in her subject. I don't know why, but I sensed that she really cared about her work, her discipline.'

Maureen nodded. She had heard that about other neurologists. She always felt they must be quite special in a way, having to constantly work with people in pain, or people facing progressive disability and sometimes with little hope of any kind of recovery, more often a slow progression towards greater disability. 'Sounds like she made a really big and positive impression.'

'I came away feeling that I could go back to her when I needed to.'

'Something about her which makes that feel easy for you.'

'Hmm. But I am going back in four weeks. She talked about what can be done to ease the pain, and ways to manage my activity to minimise the tiredness. That was helpful. Things I'd never thought of. And she also told me more about some of the other complications that can arise with MS, none too pleasant.' Gerry's lips tightened. 'Seems to depend on what areas of the spinal cord are affected, what signals are disrupted. Bladder, bowel problems – they don't sound too good. And it can affect how you think, memory. But not everyone gets everything. She really was at pains to point that out.'

'Hmm, a lot to have to come to terms with?'

Gerry nodded. 'Yes, oh, and I asked her about cannabis, you know? Read about how people find it really helpful? Used it a little myself in the past. Apparently it can ease the pain. She wouldn't encourage me in this, said that professionally she couldn't, but it was up to me. She said that there were trials going on looking at its effectiveness. She said that personally she hoped that it would become medically available, that part of the problem, if it was shown to be helpful, was that there was little control over dose when you smoked it yourself. She sounded quite open and progressive in her thinking, but avoided saying anything that suggested I should go off and start smoking it again! And that's understandable.' He smiled. Maureen smiled back.

'I'm just feeling very aware of what a difference it makes when you at least have an idea as to what's going on, you know? I mean, when you're in pain, tired and you know something's wrong, but you don't really understand what it is, it must add to the anxiety?'

'And to the depression. But the way she explained it just made it somehow seem less scary. I mean, it's still horrible to think about, but I'm clearer about what it is now. And I've got a lot of ideas to try.'

'Mhmm, exercise, do you mean?'

'Yes, and being careful with movement, and not overdoing it. Talked about how muscles weaken or can go into spasm easily. Also the need to keep my mind alert and active. There can be cognitive problems and, while I haven't experienced them, I need to keep my mind active. She also mentioned diet, that there are some things to avoid, and some supplements that some people find helpful. She said that there are no guarantees but some things work for some people. I asked about alcohol, and, well, she said it depended on quantity but high intake wasn't helpful, would just complicate some of the symptoms, which makes sense.'

Maureen momentarily went back to her last supervision session. 'So that's not an option then!'

'No, and I am aware that it had become a feature of my life, but I do need to watch that. But she said it is about experimenting and seeing what seems to have an effect. We ended up talking a bit more about the cannabis option. She explained how the government are appraising this, or at least some part of the Department of Health is. And that medical trials are ongoing.'

'So, you have come away with some tangible ideas to follow through and a strong sense of reassurance that you are in the hands of someone who knows what they are talking about.' Maureen saw no need to say anything more about alcohol. How often that happened. Spend time on something in supervision, and the next session the client has resolved it for themselves, or already processed something.

It does seem to happen sometimes that a topic or issue worked through in supervision, to prepare the counsellor to work more effectively and authentically at the next session, turns out to be something that the client has already found a solution to. I remember a supervisor of mine who always said that work done in supervision was work done for the client – the implication being that somehow processing and clarification in supervision can in some way impact on the client. While this might be considered too fantastic and implausible to some, I have experienced it occurring often and have heard others say the same. Perhaps the ancient axiom 'energy follows thought' has a significance for therapists that means the psychological dynamics of the therapeutic relationship extend beyond the hourly session and the consulting room. It is an area requiring research.

Gerry nodded. 'Yes. And she has put me on some medication to help slow the progression of the disease.'

'Mhmm.'

'And I told her about how I had overdone it in the pool, and she confirmed that it was very likely that it had triggered that flare-up. She suggested a little and often, to keep the muscles mobile but without so much stress on them. She said that there were a variety of medications that really did help, that there had been a lot of developments in treatment over the years.'

'Mhmm.'

'But I don't want to take anything unless I really have to. She also said that they can prescribe steroids, but that brings with it another set of side-effects. It's a jungle. Whichever way you turn there is risk of damage. But I guess it's about coping as best as I can and learning to accept that there will be times when I will need the medication and I should be grateful for it. But that doesn't come easy to me. I don't like drugs, of having to take chemicals if I can avoid it.'

'You'd rather keep away from them; it's going to be difficult accepting and being grateful for them.'

Gerry replied, 'Yeah, makes you wonder what it was like in the past, you know, all the pain people must have suffered with no relief. I guess they just got drunk, or maybe some herbal potion or other helped, I don't know.'

'Must have been awful. As you say, it makes you think, and appreciate what we have now.'

'Yes, but she has persuaded me to take one particular medication to try to limit the impact of the disease, even though I'm not in pain at the moment. They have a range of drugs that they can try and she has prescribed one of them. I expressed my concerns, and she did listen but she was quite firm. She's a small woman, but she was very assertive. I don't think I'd want to get the wrong side of her, you know? But I felt I could trust her and she persuaded me to take this stuff. Anyway, there may be no immediate effect, but I have to persevere. However, if I get problems with side-effects I need to get in touch and she will arrange for the GP to prescribe an alternative. Apparently some medications disagree more with some people than others.'

'So, treatment to minimise the damage, and a few ideas as to what you can do to combat it as well.'

'Yes, oh, and there was someone from an MS support network there, giving out leaflets in the waiting room. Apparently, they have this sort of stand – well, table – with information when the consultant holds her outpatient clinics. So I had a chat with a woman who was there and there is apparently a local group, and she has given me details of an organisation to join which acts as a kind of lobbying group as well as offering ideas, information, support, social get-togethers for people suffering with MS. I may go along sometime to see what it's like.'

'Meet other people, maybe get some ideas, and I guess be with people who understand what it is like first hand.'

'Yes, though I know part of me is reluctant in case I find it depressing, seeing what happens to people. The lady said they were a jolly lot but I can kind of imagine everyone being depressed. But maybe I'm just being a bit negative. I guess I need to go along and find out.'

Maureen nodded and Gerry found himself not knowing quite what to say next. He felt he had said what he wanted to say about the appointment with the consultant. Yes, it had been reassuring. He was going to see her again as much to monitor the situation as anything else. She explained that they would continue doing further tests. He'd explained about it at work and they had been good about him taking the time out to go to the hospital without having to take annual leave. He still felt they didn't really understand, but at least they were being supportive of him, so that felt positive.

'So,' he finally said, 'I'm not sure what to say next.'

'Mhmm, run out of things to say.'

Gerry sat and thought about it. He didn't really feel he had more to say. He felt that he was in safe hands and it felt like as one door closed another had opened. 'I kind of feel that the counselling came at just the right time and has really helped me in a way prepare myself for seeing the consultant. I don't think I'd have reacted the same if I'd seen her, say, three months ago. I think I was too full of my own self-pity, too fearful, too self-isolating to have really heard what the consultant said. And I don't think I'd have been able to feel I could take some responsibility for my own treatment, for kind of self-managing the condition, which I feel I can do now. So I'm really grateful for that. And though it isn't something we've kind of directly talked about, I've changed and benefited from it.'

'I sense you have changed a great deal, but you're the one who really knows what that feels like. To me, you seem more accepting and more ready and willing to make the best of things.'

'Before I couldn't see beyond my own wallowing in self-pity.'

'And maybe that was necessary too.'

'Do you think so?'

Oops, thought Maureen, now I have to explain myself. Still, it's the last session and we are moving out of therapeutic emphasis to a more conversational style (although she thought that often a bit more conversation could be valuable for some clients). 'It's maybe a stage, a very human reaction to the shock of the possibility of having a progressive disability diagnosed, and to the pain. I kind of sense that maybe you've given yourself a hard time of it, but it is just another part of the process.'

'Not a very healthy part, though.'

'No, but sometimes we do turn in on ourselves to cope – well, you know that – it's just ...' Maureen was aware she was getting lost in her own sentence, '... well, there's a huge sense of loss and fear and they are things that we feel sorry about.'

'Hmm.' Gerry wasn't convinced. He didn't like how he had been and the impact it had had on the family. But he wasn't going to debate the point. He knew how he felt about things and he didn't feel he needed to justify them to anyone else.

An example of Gerry trusting his own internal locus of evaluation. He doesn't feel a need to have to get approval from someone else, or change someone else's view to his own to feel comfortable with his own evaluation. He can accept his own perspective.

'It suddenly feels odd, like I know we are going to end soon, but wondering how to fill the time.'

'Like waiting to say goodbye to someone who is about to leave, but the taxi hasn't arrived yet?' Maureen wasn't sure where that image came from, but it just sort of came out.

'Something like that. Look, I want to say thank you. I really do appreciate your time and your skills. You've turned me around, and I'm really not sure exactly how. I can't say you did something specific, or said something that I can point to and say, that was it. But I am different. I have changed. And I feel ready to move on. I'm going to get support from the consultant when I see her, though I'm sure I'll see other members of her team as well. I feel like I'm reconnected with my family. The remission is good, well, I guess that's not the right word to call it. I gather that MS can be benign, maybe it will settle for me, but I know as well that it can get progressively worse, sometimes gradually, sometimes in fits and starts. I know that even though I feel good now the possibility of it flaring up again is in the background, and maybe it always will be even if there has been little damage, or the damage is contained and controlled. It's strange, but I feel kind of fascinated by it now, I want to understand more. Like something is happening to my body and I want to be more aware of it, want to somehow, I don't know, engage with it. I mean, shit, it's my body. I think that's partly me, but also the effect of the consultant. She seemed so enthusiastic – that's probably not the right word, but you know what I mean.'

'Sounds like she has a real sense of vocation for her speciality and it's fired your curiosity.'

'Very much.'

'Well, it seems like you've told me what you feel you have got out of counselling, and you have ideas for your steps forward, you have support out there and the possibility of getting involved with that local group. I'd like to say something as well.'

Gerry looked slightly surprised.

'Well, I've really valued the time we have had here, Gerry, and it has touched me enormously seeing and hearing about your struggle, and the moments that touched you deeply, of your past and of your anxieties and hopes for the future. It's felt real, it's felt like therapy, and I can honestly say that I've learned a lot about MS and the effects it can have, and the process of coming to terms with it.'

Gerry nodded, and could feel his eyes watering.

'And yes, I want to say that I really value your sensitivity, and I appreciate as well how difficult that is for you at times. It's a great quality to have. So, I feel privileged meeting you and I really do wish you well for the future.' As she spoke Maureen was feeling deeply affected. She liked Gerry. She was so pleased that he had moved on from where he was at the start of the sessions.

'Thanks. I wasn't expecting that. You really mean it, don't you?'

Maureen nodded. 'I try not to say things I don't mean. I meant what I said. It's about being real, allowing what is present for me to be present in this therapeutic relationship. It can feel risky, but it's normally a more satisfying way to be.'

'I'm kind of interested in how you work, your philosophy of counselling. Are there any books on it?'

'Yes. I work in what is called a "person-centred" way. It is an approach that was founded by an American called Carl Rogers. He wrote a number of books and you can usually find some of them in bookstores in the counselling section.'

'Is there one that you would recommend?'

Now, thought Maureen, here's an interesting conundrum. How to recommend a Carl Rogers book without being directive! 'Well, I guess it depends maybe on how technical you want to be. There's something called *The Carl Rogers Reader*, a collection of his writings, including excerpts from books. That's worth looking out for. Some people prefer his earlier writings, others his later ones, often depending on their own perception of the approach.'

'OK, *The Carl Rogers Reader*. Was he the author then?'

'The collection was put together by two people, Kirschenbaum and Henderson.'

'How do you spell, what did you say ...?'

'Kirschenbaum, I think that's K-I-R-S-C-H-E-N-B-A-U-M. Oh and Brian Thorne has written a book on Rogers' life, I think just called *Carl Rogers*.'

'Thanks. I appreciate that. OK, so, time to go. Thanks again.'

'I'm glad it has been of help. Take care. I hope things work out well for you.'

'And for you too.' As he said it Gerry realised that he knew absolutely nothing about Maureen. All he knew was that she was a counsellor that listened to him. He smiled as he shook her hand. 'You know, I was just thinking that I know nothing about you, and you know so much about me.'

Maureen nodded and with a slightly wicked tone to her voice replied, 'That's therapy.'

The relationship ended in smiles, and both felt a bit of a lump in their throats. Two people had met, one the client, the other the counsellor. Both had been changed by the experience.

Points for discussion

- What is present for you at the moment of finishing reading? Discuss the impact of the dialogue on you.
- Was everything addressed in supervision that you felt should have been addressed? If not, what was missing?
- How would you define empathy in your own words, and what are your thoughts on the discussion between Maureen and Donna regarding 'empathic understanding' and 'empathic appreciation'?
- Define intuition. What role does it have in person-centred practice and how might it be linked to person-centred theory?
- Counsellors often talk about beginnings, middles and endings. What is the therapeutic value of honouring the new beginning as a feature of the ending process?
- As sessions draw to a final conclusion the dialogue can become more conversational. What might a more conversational style of counselling have to offer a client?
- Was there anything that you might have wanted to include in that final session had you been the counsellor?
- Write your own notes for the counselling session.

Gerry reflects on his experience of counselling

Gerry left that final session feeling quite emotional. He had really come to like Maureen and those sessions had become quite an important part of his week. At the same time, he also felt good that he was moving on. He saw the ending very much as a new beginning, and that was both exciting and tinged with some anxiety.

It had been helpful to have someone to talk things through with. It had been a long wait to see the consultant, and having seen her he had felt reassured and it had taken a lot of the anxiety out. Up until then he hadn't really been clear as to what could be done, how bad it might become.

His mood still fluctuated. He found it frustrating on bad days not to be able to move as freely as he would want. He understood that there could be lengthy periods of remission, but then it could flare up. He had felt supported by Maureen. She really cared, really listened. That had felt good. She seemed solid, quietly reassuring, not because of being an expert on MS or anything like that, he knew that she wasn't, but just her presence as a person had really helped. He couldn't really explain it, but it had left him with a sense of how helpful counselling could be and he hoped that, if things got on top of him again, he would be able to ask for similar help once more. He didn't want to overly rely on it. But it had helped.

He knew he had an uncertain future ahead of him. The list of possible complications associated with MS was daunting. But he felt he was surrounded by people who cared for him, who loved him, who wanted to help him. His eyes watered and he felt a lump in his throat as he thought about it. He knew he'd battle on; he owed that to his family, and to himself. He knew there'd be times when he'd probably feel too tired to want to fight it, when he might need to lean on others to get him through, but he'd try and avoid that if he could. It was something that you tended to think happened to other people, you didn't think – well, he hadn't thought – of developing a progressive disability. Certainly brought life into a sharper focus.

He thought back over the sessions. He couldn't remember much of what had happened. Certainly the early sessions, he didn't think he was in place to really take much on board at all. And yet one moment stood out, well, not one, it had happened more than once. He wished now he'd mentioned it before he'd left. It was the eye contact. There were moments when he had looked across the room into Maureen's eyes, and she had held his gaze. They had been so incredibly powerful. He couldn't really describe the effect but somehow, in spite of all the talking, they were the moments that stood out for him. He had felt connected, but not just to Maureen, to himself as well. In those moments he had felt strangely more present. He couldn't really explain it. Ah well, he thought, I know who to read about it. Maybe that chap she talked about at the end would have the answer, what was his name? Oh yes, Roger something … no, Rogers. He'd look out for him.

Maureen assesses her experience of being Gerry's counsellor

Maureen had really valued her work with Gerry and it had certainly opened her up to the challenge of empathising with someone suffering physical pain, and who faced a future with the very real possibility of progressive disability. She had found it difficult and it had drawn awkward and uncomfortable feelings into her awareness. She had found herself wanting to move him on, wanting things to improve. She was glad that the symptoms had eased. She felt sad that the relationship had ended but at the same time she experienced a certain sense of timeliness about it. It had acted as a kind of bridge between where Gerry had been in his process to where he now was, and what that meant in terms of him perhaps being able to better use the advice given by the consultant.

She wondered what might have stood out for Gerry. She remembered him saying that he couldn't point to any one thing that had made the difference. She wasn't surprised. It could happen, but often it was simply the process of being in therapeutic relationship, of experiencing contact with another person who is seeking to offer authenticity, empathy and unconditional positive regard, and experiencing their presence. But there had been moments that had touched her deeply. His daughter wanting to push the wheelchair. That had seemed such a ... well, such a *human* moment. Utterly spontaneous. How we need those. She could feel emotional just thinking about it. And his son wanting a red one, what was it, something about a Ferrari engine. Wonderful stuff.

But the moments that stood out for her were moments of eye contact. There had been a few and some had seemed incredibly profound. It was like they met but it was more than a meeting. It was as though in that moment there was a knowing, an understanding, and it was characterised by mutuality, and yet she did not know quite what it was she had been left knowing or understanding. She wouldn't forget those. Funny, I didn't mention them to Gerry, or to Donna, come to think of it. Maybe I will in the next supervision. Or will I? The more she thought about it, the more she felt she probably wouldn't. They somehow seemed too precious to share, somehow deeply affirming in a way that might be lost if talked about. She wanted to just hold her memory of an experience that in truth she couldn't really put into words without losing something of the experience. It felt good to know those moments had happened and could happen. Moments of spontaneous connection. She wondered what Gerry had experienced in them. Oh well, I'll never know now. But there was something about those moments that gave her goosebumps when she thought about them.

PART 2

The reality of mobility loss

CHAPTER 5

Setting the scene

Pauline has been suffering from MS since her twenties. She is now in her early fifties and is really struggling to walk. She sits a lot and has got lower back pain, and her muscles are not responding well, her central nervous system now being damaged to the point that she finds it impossible at times to co-ordinate her muscle activity. Pauline finds it very difficult to maintain her balance; she has to sit a lot and often be helped up. Sometimes she has to stay in bed.

Her condition has recently deteriorated. Her better days do not allow her much movement, although she can get around the house, into the garden and out to the car.

Pauline's partner of many years, Diana, is extremely supportive of her. They live in a bungalow that has been adapted for Pauline's needs. She remains cheerful in spite of her difficulties. Over the years she has been on various medications to try to hold back the development of the condition. They helped to some degree but the progression has continued relentlessly. Life has been a series of struggles, clinging to personal freedoms until the last moment – for instance, having to give up work, which was a major blow to Pauline. However, she has been active in a MS support group, although there have been times when she has not been able to attend. She found this hard to come to terms with.

The pain in her back makes it difficult for her to type – she used to do a lot of secretarial work. She does not want to stop this but is finding that she is typing increasingly slowly. She has thought about a voice-activated system but feels she does not want to lose her typing skills, not just yet anyway.

At a recent consultation with her GP, Pauline broke down in tears. This was unusual and the GP was concerned. After a lengthy consultation and discussion on the subject, Pauline agreed to see a counsellor. She did not want to go to the surgery counsellor as she felt she wanted to see someone who had an appreciation of MS. She had contacted a local disability information centre and they had put her in touch with a counsellor who, fortunately, lived fairly close to her. He had agreed to visit her at home, for which she was extremely grateful.

Counselling session 1: getting to know the client

Pauline was in a lot of pain but was determined she would see the counsellor. She had spoken to him on the phone and had felt extremely comfortable talking to him. He seemed to appreciate something of her difficulties. She didn't want to have to start explaining her symptoms and history, and educating the counsellor in MS and disability. She had had so many different consultants and junior specialists over the years, and she was fed up with going over it all time and again.

She was grateful that he was coming to see her at home. It would make it a lot more easy for her, and would mean that it wouldn't tie Diana up taking her and bringing her back. Pauline used to drive but now she found it too difficult. She could not trust the reactions of her feet on the foot pedals. There had been discussions in the past about having a purposely adapted car, but her hands weren't too good either, strange sensations leaving her struggling to grip the steering wheel. She knew she couldn't cope with foot pedals and so there wasn't much that she could be offered. It was difficult enough to get in and out of a car, let alone drive one.

She had told the counsellor – whose name was Jim – to press the intercom button when he arrived and she would let him in. She had an electronic control system for the door which was a godsend. When Diana was out she couldn't always get to the door in time to let in anyone who called. She had found it hard to accept, at first, but she realised she needed it when an old friend who she hadn't seen for a long time called. She had been in the area and just dropped by, but because she didn't get any response she left. In fact, Pauline had heard her knock but just wasn't mobile enough to get to the door in time.

She heard the buzzer go. In fact, Diana had insisted on being there the first session to let Jim in, so she had gone to the door.

'Hello, I'm Jim. You must be Pauline.'

'Actually, no, I'm her partner, Diana.'

'Oh, right, hi, pleased to meet you.' Jim reached out and shook her hand.

'Come on in. Pauline's expecting you. She's through in the front room. Go on through and turn left.'

Jim walked along the hall and turned left as he had been advised. It felt warm. There was a dark maroon carpet on the floor and a kind of light pink finish on the walls. There were a number of small paintings as well. He turned and walked into the front room. Pauline was sitting in a chair to the left. 'Hi, I'm Jim. Good to meet you.'

'Good to meet you too. Please, come in and sit down. It's so good of you to come and see me here. Makes it so much easier for me.'

'Yes, I'm sure it does. It's quite handy my being fairly close.'

'Do you want anything to drink?'

'Thanks but no. I'm fine, but please, go ahead if you want something.'

'No, I'm fine.'

Diana popped her head round the door. 'I'll leave you two to it then. I'll be in the kitchen.'

'Thanks. See you later.'

Counselling a person in their own home can raise all kinds of issues: will they be interrupted (doorbells, other people in the house, telephone); how appropriate will the seating be (the counsellor may find themselves disappearing into a deep, soft sofa); how confidential will it be if others are in the home; do you accept a drink which can then delay the start of the session?

Other issues that might need considering with particular clients is how safe will it be for the counsellor? For home visits, particularly to begin with, it is worth ensuring somebody knows you are there and that they expect you to call at the end of the session to let them know all is OK.

Jim felt a little tense as he sat on the settee opposite Pauline. She clearly had an adapted chair, presumably to help her get in and out of it. He was seated about six feet away from her and was conscious of the distance. He generally sat much closer to clients. He had glanced round the room to see if there were any other chairs that he might move closer, but they had higher seats and he felt that sitting above and looking down on his client wasn't going to be too helpful. He decided to note his thoughts but not comment on them.

'So, how can I help, what do you want to get from counselling?' Jim didn't start talking about what counselling was all about. He preferred to let the client have the space to take their own direction right from the start of the session. He would say something later if the issue arose.

'Not sure, really. I had counselling a long while back, but not to do with my MS. That was around my sexuality. But that was a long time ago.'

Jim nodded. 'So you have an idea what counselling is about.'

'Yes, although I guess times have changed somewhat. But, yes, I know it's confidential and all that.'

'Mhmm, yes, I do offer confidential counselling. I do want you to feel able to talk about whatever is present for you.' Jim said a little about the possible limits to confidentiality and Pauline felt OK with that. 'Yes,' she responded, 'but I don't think I'm going to commit a terrorist outrage, and if I was, I don't think I'd be telling you about it first.'

Jim smiled. 'No, but we have to mention it. The issue that is often more likely is around child protection.'

'Hmm. Could have done with that when I was younger.'

Jim realised that he had become suddenly more alert. 'You had a difficult time?'

'Understatement. But I worked on that in the past. I guess I experienced neglect as a child. Bullied at school. Seemed to be dismissed by my parents who thought I was just whining about life, you know, looking for reasons not to go to school. But that was a long time ago. Then I started to get tingling sensations and tiredness, and headaches, the usual symptoms, that was in my mid-twenties. By then I had realised I was lesbian and fortunately had formed a lot of good friendships. People were very supportive. My family didn't really understand; they've come to terms with it now but it took them a long while. That hurt a lot.'

'Yeah, must have been very painful.' Jim really felt a sense of how that must have felt, not being accepted for who you were by those closest to you.

'Once the symptoms started, well, life started to become a struggle, physical, well, and mental struggle. Just got progressively worse over the years. A few remissions. It sort of worsened in stages?'

Jim nodded. 'Mhmm, in steps.'

'I didn't understand at first, but I soon came to realise what effect it was having.'

Jim nodded. 'Not something you can really understand to begin with, but you soon discover what limitations it can cause.'

'So many things I couldn't do. I wanted to do them, but it was the pain. The headaches were bad, but the tiredness, that just floored me at times. Some days though I was OK. Just never knew. In fact, at times I went months without it being really bad, and then it would set on again. So I did get to do things, you know, and getting away on holidays and generally travelling, but it really started to limit me in my thirties. Didn't stop me with work and I had a social life and things like that, but it was cramping my style. Never felt very confident, always felt awkward, and put it down to my condition, you know? Now, well, I've got a tough choice, and that's what's been upsetting me.' She took a deep breath. 'The day that's been out there, waiting for me suddenly seems all too close.'

'And that's what you mentioned on the phone, yes?'

Pauline tightened her lips. 'Yes.' She knew she wanted to talk it through with someone, somebody who would tell her what to do. Diana was good, she loved her, she was such a comfort and her madcap humour really helped enormously, but she did seem to have her own agenda which seemed to be based around encouraging Pauline to accept the reality of her situation. Pauline didn't want to do that.

Jim waited. He felt that it was Pauline's call. She knew what she wanted to talk about and he didn't want to introduce a specific focus. Rather, it felt more appropriate to allow her to find her own words, in her own time, and to tell him what she wanted him to hear, to understand, to appreciate.

Person-centred counselling is a non-directive, therapeutic discipline. It is important to allow the client to feel free to find their own words, their own direction. This way of relating needs to be introduced at the start of counselling, setting the tone and helping to inform the expectations of the client.

'The MS has got a lot worse these last 12 months. I've had steroids a few times but can't keep on them, too much risk, but you know that. And I've used cannabis on and off over the years. Sometimes it's helped, not always.'

Jim nodded. He'd mentioned on the phone that he had an understanding of the effects of MS from his involvement in offering counselling at a pain clinic in another part of the country, prior to moving to where he now lived.

'Yes, but it's a bugger when whatever you take for relief you know is adding risk elsewhere.'

Pauline took a deep breath, which wasn't a comfortable thing to do. As her ribs expanded she could feel the discomfort intensify in her back. She tended to shallow breathe. She knew that wasn't good for her, but it was more comfortable. She was feeling stiff. She pulled her shoulders back slightly and moved them forward a bit, turning slightly in the chair to try and unlock her back a little. She took it very carefully. She knew from experience the effects of sudden movement – could leave her in pain for quite some while. It wasn't worth the risk, and particularly not today which wasn't too good.

Jim noticed her wince. 'Painful to move, yeah, bad day?' He felt sympathetic. Yes, he knew that counsellors were supposed to do empathy, not sympathy, but he was human and he was in front of someone in pain and suffering. Yes, he felt sorry for her, damned sorry. But he knew as well that he wanted to understand and appreciate what she was experiencing, not just how he felt about it.

'Not one of my best. Anyway, so, where were we?'

'Painkillers, steroids, cannabis, side-effects.'

'Oh yes. Well, so, I have to try and be careful. I have to keep taking medication, I'd be a lot worse without it, I'm sure, not that I'm that flexible, although I probably have more movement than I can manage.'

Jim guessed she meant that the movement was restricted by the pain. 'Pain barrier?'

'Yes. Good way of putting it.'

He'd made the comment often. Some people had greater tolerance to pain and could push that barrier, others didn't. It wasn't a matter of being weak-willed although he had met people who seemed to just push on in spite of pain. Pain is very personal. Jim knew that. No one can fully understand the pain of another. Even if they have a similar condition, it won't necessarily be experienced in exactly the same way. People could become almost attached to their pain; it became so much a part of their experience. Sometimes at the pain clinic he had worked with people where there was virtually no apparent cause of pain, no physical disease, and yet somehow their brain was receiving signals along the central nervous system that was triggering a pain event. It could be so restrictive, but with MS, of course, it wasn't simply pain; there was actual damage to the central nervous system and loss of control in some areas of the body.

Jim nodded and waited.

Pauline was pondering on what Jim had said. 'And it's not just a barrier to me, you know, I mean a barrier stopping me do things. It puts up a barrier between me and other people.'

'I can appreciate that, people kind of back away, is that what you mean?'

'Yes. People find it hard to cope with pain, particularly when they haven't experienced it for themselves. They feel, I don't know, but you kind of find out who your friends are. Some people can cope with it, they can somehow sit with you when the times are tough, but others don't want to know. And not just the pain, the disability too. I've had friends that I've really known well, but they've kind of dropped away as my disability has worsened. People I would never have expected that reaction from. And others have stuck with me, through thick and thin. Strange, but not strange. But you find out who your friends are.'

'And that can be . . .' Jim was about to say 'distressing', but realised it was an assumption, although highly likely to be accurate.

'. . . hard to accept.' Pauline finished his sentence for him. 'Hard to accept. I mean, I had a friend, Marjorie, we were really good friends, went about together a lot and I felt she really did understand my difficulties, you know? Right up to about five years ago, and then suddenly she stopped visiting me. Still don't know why. It felt somehow awkward a couple of times and then, that was that. Never heard any more. Not even a Christmas card. I sent for a couple of years but the second year it came back – not known at this address. I don't know what happened, but the awkwardness, I don't know, something happened, and I kind of sense it was to do with me, my worsening condition.'

'That something about your condition getting worse got to her in some way, for some reason, and she stopped coming.'

'I'll probably never know why,' Pauline paused, 'never know why.' She had memories of Marjorie, how they'd have laughs and reminisce about the past. She'd got married and had a family. She never said anything about finding Pauline's sexuality an issue. It wasn't something that had been a factor, she felt, in their relationship. But she had seemed to back away. And she wasn't the only one. People from where she had worked as well.

'It wasn't just Marjorie. When I had to give up work, around the same time actually, people were saying how they'd keep in touch but hardly anyone has. I worked for that company for ten years, you know. OK, people came and went. But some people I knew there for a long while. But who stayed in touch? Well, there's Lucy and there's Barry, who's gay and just so camp! I love him dearly and, well, in a way he makes up for everyone who hasn't kept in touch. He's just so outrageous, so outrageous, and, well, so much I can say about him.' She knew she was smiling, just at the mention of him and the thought of him, coming in, regaling her with his various exploits and wit.

'He's really important, the way you speak of him.' Jim was aware of smiling too. Pauline had a lovely smile and it felt kind of infectious.

'Yes. It's strange, but not strange. People either can and do stick with me, or they vanish. It really feels all or nothing sometimes. And that hurts. But the people who are friends are good friends, and that's important to me. Really important.'

Jim nodded. 'Yes, important for you to have friends, really good friends.'

Pauline moved again in the chair; she was locking up once more and needed to free her back. The cushion that she had behind her had slipped down and it was uncomfortable; she liked it a little higher.

Jim noticed that she seemed to be trying to manipulate it back up, but couldn't.
'Can I do something?'
'Can you just lift the cushion up a bit, thanks, trying to shift it without moving too much.'
Jim got up and lifted the cushion back to where Pauline wanted it.
'Thanks. On days like this I don't move more than I have to.'
Jim had sat back down.

> Jim offering to do something is a conveying of empathy as well as being practical. He is showing he is aware of what is present for Pauline and offering to help. It all helps in the relationship and trust-building process.

'You find it better to be still, but then you lock up.'
'That's the problem. Not all days are as bad as this, though sometimes they are worse.'
The session continued with Pauline giving Jim a bit more of her history. She was describing how her condition had worsened over the years and how it had been difficult to accept having to give up her work. She'd gone down to part-time for a while but that had become too much as well.
'Everything's such a bloody battle when you're disabled. Everything. People park in the disabled bays and then get pissed off with you when you try to get them to move; they barge into you, even when they see you are struggling when you're walking along the street. Not being "normal". Sometimes I hate so-called "normal people". What the hell do they know about what I'm feeling, I'm experiencing? People talk over and around you, "the does she take sugar" syndrome, still happens. When I've been bad, visitors talk to Di about me. She's good, steers them to talk to me. It's cruelty, it relegates you to feeling like a non-person.' She looked at Jim. 'I don't expect you to understand. It's being made to feel less of a person because of how you move, or can't move, your body. I want to fucking scream at them sometimes, "For fuck's sake, I'm a person like you. I don't want to be like this, but I can't help it. I'm a person in here, like you, a woman. Talk to me, relate to me." Just gets to me sometimes.'
'Rage at people, at . . .'
'. . . at everything. Benefits. Bloody hell. Do they believe you? Always struggling to get what you deserve and then being terrified that they'll take it away again.' She paused, before continuing. 'And you know, the one thing more than any that really gets my goat, normal people who use the disabled loo and cause you to have to wait. For fuck's sake, at least I can stand OK on good days, but sometimes, you know, keeping your balance and bursting for a pee, and then they don't like it when you glare at them, they make some rude comment or other. Maybe it's better when you're in a wheelchair, I don't know, maybe people are more accepting of your disability. Guess I've got that one to discover for myself.'

'I can't pretend to say I understand, but I can imagine, yeah, always being made to feel different and less of a person, what that must do to you. Shit. Fucking nightmare.'

'And now comes the next battle.'

Jim nodded. Yes, he thought, for many the hardest battle of all.

'So, what do I do? I mean, I have to keep walking, I have to keep using my muscles, I can't afford to let them go to waste. I can't do that, can I?'

Jim wanted to say 'no you can't', but he restrained himself and kept to his empathy, seeking to clarify his understanding. 'That's the dilemma, you can't risk letting your muscles go to waste by not using them.'

Pauline was looking down. She hadn't done that at all during the session. 'No, I mustn't let that happen. Somehow, I've got to keep going, got to keep walking. Can't stop that, mustn't stop that, but sometimes, it is so painful. It's excruciating and, well, hard to describe. It can come on, like sharp, hot pain; at other times it just stays like an intense grating ache, and sometimes both. On really bad days it doesn't matter whether I move or not, the pain's there. I have to take the painkillers. It's a bugger, it really is.'

'Yeah, got to keep walking but it's so damned excruciating. A complete and utter bugger.' Jim spoke slowly, really acknowledging his appreciation of what Pauline was saying.

Pauline heard Jim and stayed silent. Did he really understand what she was going through? Did anyone? No, that was silly, she knew people through the MS network who knew, course they did. But what about Jim? So he'd worked with people in pain, but had he experienced pain? Did he *really* know, *really* understand? She felt he kind of did; at least, he seemed to appreciate what she was saying and how she was saying it. But did he understand what it felt like, really felt like? She felt she needed to know.

'Have you ever experienced severe pain?'

'Like you experience?'

'Well, yes, but any severe pain?'

'No. Does that sound strange?'

No. I mean, you seem to appreciate what I am saying, but I'm wondering how much you really understand what it is like.'

'Not from my own personal experience, no. But I have been touched by what you have said and while I don't, can't, feel your physical pain, I can get a kind of sense of the feelings you have towards it.'

'I'm tired of it.' Pauline spoke in a very tired kind of way.

'Tired of . . . all the pain?'

'The pain, the struggle, the tiredness, the . . . everything.'

'Yeah, tired of all of it.'

'Yeah.' Pauline went silent. Yes, tired of it, tired of it all. She found herself sitting without thinking at all. She was feeling blank, or rather, she wasn't feeling at all, or thinking. She just sat staring ahead of herself.

Jim sat with the silence. It felt like a 'there's nothing more to say' kind of silence. So he respected that and maintained his empathy for Pauline's silence through his own communication of silence back to her. They continued to sit, and a minute or two passed.

Pauline moved her back slightly and snorted, tightening her lips as she did so. 'No good me sitting here feeling sorry for myself.'

'You don't want to feel sorry for yourself?'

'Can't afford to. Can't let myself slip into that too often. Doesn't do me any good, or anyone else for that matter, particularly Di. She's so good for me, to me. Without her . . .' Pauline's voice trailed off and Jim noticed her eyes welling up with tears.

'Yeah, without her . . .'

Jim empathises with the unanswered question, allowing Pauline to know that it was heard but leaving her free to answer it either to herself, verbally or both, if she wishes.

'I'm getting all emotional today, aren't I?' Pauline had got a tissue and was dabbing at her eyes. 'And I'm not really talking about the real issue.'

'Mhmm, but maybe you are talking about other important aspects to it all. But yes, I appreciate you aren't talking about the issue you mentioned on the phone.'

Pauline did feel emotional and yet she felt calm as well. She was also aware of coming over extremely tired, which was not unusual. She took a sip of water.

'I feel like my concentration's beginning to go. Gets like that sometimes. The pain saps my energy and I can struggle to keep focused. I can drift off quite easily sometimes, watching a film, you know, and I'm often having to ask Di what's happened, what's going on. I lose the plot. It's so frustrating and yet sometimes I'm so tired I haven't even enough energy to feel frustrated.'

'You really don't have much in reserve, too much concentration and you drift and lose the plot. You feel you want to draw the session to a close? We are nearly up to time, well, getting close.'

Pauline nodded. 'Yes, can we? Let's stop here. It's been good talking to you. You do listen, don't you? I really feel like you've listened to me with all my ramblings and I appreciate that.'

'I'm glad you felt listened to because, yes, I was and am listening. I do want to appreciate and understand what you are experiencing and describing. It is only the first session but I feel I've got to know you, got a sense of who you are. So, are you happy to continue and, if so, how often?'

'I think it needs to be weekly, at least to begin with. I seem to have avoided what I need to talk about this week, but I'll try not to next week.'

'I guess you'll bring to the session what you feel to be most pressing and what you feel most able to talk about.'

'Sometimes what's most pressing isn't what I feel most able to talk about, though.'

'No. I can appreciate that.' He paused, hesitant as to whether to say anything more or continue with the ending.

'So, same time next week, is that OK?'

'Sure.'

They had already agreed a fee over the phone and Pauline had it in an envelope – cash – which she handed to Jim as he got up. She confirmed what they had agreed and he thanked her.

'I'll see you next week. You take care of yourself.'

'I'll try. Don't get too much chance of mischief!' Pauline had a slight twinkle in her eye as she spoke.

Jim smiled. He restrained from commenting back. He liked to leave clients with their own last word. 'See you next week, Pauline.' As he opened the door, Pauline called out to Diana, who came out of the kitchen.

'All finished?'

'Yes, thanks.'

'Are you coming back?'

'Yes, next week.'

'Great. I think she needs to talk to someone.' Diana had dropped her voice. 'I'm kind of too close and, well, I hope it went well.'

'I felt so but that's a question you need to ask Pauline. Anyway, bye for now.'

'Bye.'

Jim walked down the path towards his car. He had a smile on his face. He was pleased he hadn't breached confidentiality with Diana. Of course, how much she might have heard from the session – well, he didn't know, and that was for them to discuss. He didn't know how thin the walls were.

He was glad to have met Pauline. Courageous lady, he thought to himself as he opened the car door. What a life, so much pain, so much struggle. Yes, he felt he could be there for her, listen to her, give her space to think things through, be how she needed to be. Her asking him about his experience of pain was a good one. Wasn't the first time, but he had learned to be honest in those situations. Authenticity. No point in anything else. Start being evasive and, well, that's not good for the relationship and, as he knew, relationship was the key. He felt good that he and Pauline had begun to build a relationship and he was already looking forward to seeing her next week.

Meanwhile, Diana had brought Pauline a cup of tea. 'So, have you decided then?'

'Didn't talk about it. Talked about lots of things, but not that. He's a good listener, but I was flagging by the end. We'll talk more next week. Yes, I think he'll be good for me. He seems genuine enough, you know. I could see by his reactions, the expression on his face, that he was taking on board what I was saying, and I think feeling touched by it all. That was good to see. I didn't want some stony faced man sitting there staring at me for an hour! No, he seemed sensitive, genuine, open – answered a direct question about his own experience of pain. That felt good, hearing him be open about that. I've heard of counsellors who never say anything about themselves – I wouldn't want that. So, yes, it felt – feels – good. Glad he came. I think I've a lot more talking to do.' She was smiling. Yes, it had felt good. Somehow it felt a little lighter in the room.

Counselling session 2: pain and the prospect of a wheelchair explored

Jim was pulling his car up outside Pauline's house. He was a few minutes early, which he had planned for. He wanted to take that time to centre himself before starting the session. He had purposefully played some relaxing music as he had driven along. Now, he turned it off and sat back in the seat, closing his eyes. His thoughts went back to the previous session, to his feelings towards Pauline and her situation. He didn't try to make himself think or feel anything, rather he just sought to let what was present for him simply be. He felt it was important to be connected, to have a sense of what was present for him. He didn't believe in clearing his mind and feelings before a session – not that he thought you could. He felt that to be incongruent. Better to go into the session with an awareness of what is present for you. He wanted to feel he could be authentically present, which for him meant being accurately aware of his experiencing.

He took a deep breath and slowly breathed out. Yes, he thought, it's good to feel alive and to feel able to offer something of himself to others. He took another deep breath and thought of Pauline, simply holding his sense of her in his mind and his heart. He noted a feeling of warmth for Pauline. He breathed out again. He felt a certain stillness present within him. He felt ready now.

He got out of the car and headed up the path, and rang the buzzer.

'Hello, Jim here.'

'Hi, come on in.'

Jim pushed the door and went through, down the hallway and into the lounge. Pauline was sitting in her chair.

'Hi, please have a seat.'

'Thanks.' Jim sat down opposite her. He guessed that Diana was out. He said nothing; he would let Pauline tell him if it was important to her to tell him. 'So, how would you like to use our time today?'

Jim noticed Pauline take a deep breath as he finished his question, and she looked down. He sat and waited, maintaining his attention on her and his openness to his own experiencing.

An important element of effective person-centred therapy is the attitude held by the therapist. The aim is to be present, as fully present as possible. The client is the primary focus of attention and an attitude of reaching out to them is sought. Even in silence there is a quality of relatedness being established. Jim will be allowing Pauline the space she needs to find the words that she wants to say. His role is to be attentive to her process, to whatever she seeks to communicate and to his own organismic reaction – in other words, what becomes present within his own experience as a result of the sensed relatedness with his client.

Pauline could feel a tightness in her chest. That was not unusual; it came with her condition and the effect of trying not to move her back more than she had to. She was, however, having a better day and the pain had diminished and she had more movement. She knew that she must take advantage of this. She always tried to stay positive, but the pain made it so difficult. And she didn't feel so tired either. Today, though, she knew she had to start talking about the real issue, the one that had been her reason for calling Jim in the first place. Her heart was pounding, and she knew it was anxiety. She closed her eyes. Shit, she thought, this is harder than she had expected.

Jim sensed that Pauline was struggling and he knew, from that earlier telephone conversation, what her current struggle was. But he instinctively knew that she needed to find her own way of talking about it. She had managed to mention it on the phone but clearly, face to face, it was difficult.

Jim is ensuring Pauline has the space to find her own voice about the issue that has motivated her to come to counselling. He trusts that she will speak of it when she is ready, when the timing is right for her. It is the timing for the client that is therapeutically important. The person-centred counsellor trusts the process that is occurring within Pauline's field of experience.

Pauline looked up. 'Somehow it seems difficult talking about it now, and I guess I'm afraid of coming to a decision and it being the decision that I don't want to take.'

'Better not to talk about it and avoid a decision?'

'Yes, but no, I can't do that. I mean. For years I've fought to keep mobile, to keep walking and, well, on bad days I just try and avoid any movement as much as possible, you know?'

Jim nodded; he was aware that his own lips had tightened. He couldn't imagine for himself what it must be like, every day pushing yourself to walk, to get up off the bed and struggle to get to the loo, to the lounge, just around the house. Every day faced with the sure knowledge that to move meant pain, excruciating pain. He knew it was outside of his experience and he could not really understand, but he wanted to be able to communicate his understanding of whatever Pauline wanted him to grasp.

'I can't imagine what it must be like, Pauline, and yet somehow I do feel a sense of your will, your determination and your courage, and I know that that's probably not very helpful . . .' Jim realised that he was blathering on and not saying anything very helpful.

Pauline sniffed. 'I don't feel I have much courage, I just do what I do to cope, to survive, to get through, and it fucking hurts, every fucking day.' She broke down in tears. Jim looked around for tissues. Damn, he thought, there weren't any around. Stop worrying about tissues, he told himself, be there for Pauline.

'Pain, hurt, day after fucking day.' He felt for her, with her; she spoke with such sadness and he sought to reflect that in his own tone of voice. He sensed the intensity of the moment, of her emotion. He felt his own emotions as well, the impact of a fellow human being suffering in your presence. He suddenly felt very alone, wondering what on earth he had to offer her. All he could do was sit and listen. He felt suddenly very powerless. *He* was feeling powerless. For fuck's sake, he thought to himself, what have *I* got to feel powerless about. He focused back on Pauline. He knew that it was helpful to have someone with you in these dark and difficult moments. He knew he was affected by the intensity of Pauline's despair, and he was grateful. He knew that his effectiveness as a person-centred counsellor hinged very much on his being affected by his clients. Yet he also maintained his awareness of his own inner experience.

> It's an intense period, and Jim is affected by it. Is he in these moments tuning into the client's feelings, the sense of powerlessness in some way being communicated unseen into his own inner world? Or are they simply his own reactions? Are we, as human beings, carrying the potential to be more connected with each other than we might physically suppose? Such moments of deep contact can be explained in many ways. Whatever the process, they seem to be incredibly important moments.
>
> The moment probably calls for Jim to mention his experience, voicing the presence of a sensed powerlessness, thereby maybe enabling something to occur within Pauline that would have been therapeutically helpful.

Pauline felt tired of the struggle, of the daily fight, although she knew she would carry on. She rarely let her despair overcome her. Sometimes she would let it emerge when she was with Diana, but generally she kept it to herself except during those times when she just felt so low, so in need of someone to reach out to. She had a tissue tucked in at the side of the chair and she had taken it and was drying her eyes. 'Sorry.'
'You feel sorry about showing these feelings?'

> Jim acknowledging the sensed powerlessness might have enabled him to have been, in these moments, that person for Pauline to reach out to.

'I don't like to, but sometimes, they're just too much. I think of the future and I'm afraid, terrified of how it will be. I'm sure I'll get to a place one day where I want someone to take me out and shoot me, or I'll just swallow some pills or something. I don't really think like that very often, just occasionally, but only about the future. I'm not there yet. I do still enjoy life, in spite of it all. And there's Diana. She's so wonderful, so loyal, so loving, so caring. I couldn't do that to her.' She sighed, took in a deep breath and blew the air out. 'Phew, this is why I try to keep away from these feelings, they're pretty overwhelming when they're unleashed.'
'That's how you are feeling, overwhelmed?'

'Not so much now, but I was a little while ago. I kind of bottle it up and then it just gets to me. The smallest thing can set me off.'

'Some little frustration?'

She smiled. 'Yes, usually something small, like I was trying to turn on the taps in the bathroom, and sometimes Diana has forgotten and turned one off too tight and I can't turn it. Like it's hard to hold my balance. And getting things out of cupboards, high or low, they're still difficult.'

'And when you can't do the smallest thing it becomes so frustrating and it's just so upsetting, yeah, and frustrating?'

Pauline nodded. 'It's all such an effort some days and part of me feels, "Is it worth it?", while another part of me is saying, "Come on, keep on, don't give up". It's like two voices in my head. I try to keep going but some days I want to give up, and I suppose I do give up really, stay in bed later, kind of go into my shell.'

'Sometimes the voice that says "is it worth it?" dominates, yeah?'

'And that's a hard thing to admit to, but it happens. And I really don't want to be like that, but some days . . .' She paused. 'So, you see, when someone says they think I'm brave, courageous, and have a lot of determination, well, they really don't understand.'

Jim was aware he had said something like that earlier. He wasn't sure if Pauline was referring to him, but he felt he needed to make it visible to her, make it open. 'And I said it earlier, didn't I?'

'Yep.'

'Hmm. And I guess it's the mismatch then between what someone – like me – sees and experiences from the outside in contrast to what is your experience. And while I want to be open to what I experience, I really want to appreciate what is your experience. For you it isn't bravery and courage – it's a matter of survival, one day at a time, one hour at a time . . .'

A powerful response. Jim owns his error and it helps to strengthen the connection and understanding. The power of authenticity, of being able to say, as a therapist, 'I got that wrong, didn't I?', but said with a genuine desire to learn from it, can convey a great deal to the client about the sincerity of the counsellor in wanting to understand.

'Some days it's one minute at a time, Jim, it's that bad. Sometimes the pain just overwhelms me and none of the painkillers or anything touches it. Doesn't touch it. And those are the really lonely times. I can't cope with Diana being close. Just a hug is painful. I'm on my own.'

'Alone with the pain.' Jim was aware that his lips had tightened again, and he realised he was feeling very tense. His jaw was set and his back was stiff. But he felt that his own movement would detract from Pauline's focus. He decided to put up with his discomfort.

'It's like . . .' She thought about how to describe it. 'It's like molten lava inside your body, burning, burning. You know, it's like when you see a volcano blowing, spewing molten lava, it's like a burst of fiery lava kind of inside shooting down, and then my muscles can go into spasm and there's nothing I can do about it but wait. I tense up, I try not to, but I do and it doesn't help, but I can't relax. When it stops I'm tight, can't move, daren't move.'

Jim tried to imagine what it was like but knew he couldn't. He put his efforts to one side and sought to convey his empathic understanding of what Pauline was telling him.

'Burning, like molten lava, can't move, daren't move.'

'Can't, daren't, and it does pass, I know it will pass, but it just becomes my whole reality. I can only sit or lie and wait for it to pass. Sometimes Diana says I rock to and fro with it when I'm sitting. I'm not really aware that I'm doing it, but that's what I do, hunched up, just utterly, utterly locked into the pain, waiting, hoping, praying for relief.' She looked Jim strongly in the eyes. 'I pray a lot, you know, for the strength to cope.'

'You pray for the strength to cope?' Jim had been struck by her not saying she prayed for the pain to go away. But then he knew that that was like asking the impossible, so, yes, Pauline had accepted the disease but wanted strength to cope. Again, it was his view from the outside making him assume something that was not Pauline's reality.

'You sound surprised, that I pray?'

'No, my stuff, that you pray for the strength to cope, not for the pain to end.'

'It's not going to go away.' They lapsed into a momentary silence.

'I know. I realise that, Pauline, and that's the reality that you are faced with and are finding ways to cope with. And prayer plays an important part.'

Jim has taken Pauline's focus away. She was connecting with the knowing that it would never end and he has got very wordy, perhaps indicating incongruence in himself. A simple 'no, it's not going to go away' would have been more therapeutically valid.

'It does. I've learned a lot of things through this disease, a lot of things. I'm not the person I was when it started 30-odd years ago. I see life very differently, I've had to. I see things from a different perspective. Things that seem important to many people, to me, well, they're a fuss about nothing. I went through a really intolerant phase, but I realise now that was me feeling bitter and sorry for myself. That's passed. I feel sometimes like life is a great big school and I see people getting all wound up about things, but they're still in kindergarten, still playing, still experiencing, still wanting a fast-track to happiness. Not in this world, not when people die needlessly and suffer around the world from poverty. No one deserves to be pain-free while there is so much suffering, while we in the west continue to exploit the poor and the weak.' Jim could feel

Pauline's voice getting stronger as she spoke. He could feel her passion and conviction coming through.

'I really feel your passion and conviction, Pauline, no fast-track to happiness, not while people are dying needlessly.'

'I mean, and here's what gets to me, I'm totally dependent on drugs, you know? I mean, I know that when it's really bad they make fuck all difference, but otherwise, yeah, they help. I'd seize up completely without them, but, look, we've got the medication in the west to wipe out so many of the world's illnesses and infections, but do we? No. Profit rules OK? Well it's not OK. It's not OK, but I have to have their medications and they profit from my illness. It makes me fucking angry!'

Jim nodded. 'Yeah, fucking angry.'

'They make money out of my pain, of my having to take drugs that the NHS pays for. If I had my way I'd bloody well nationalise the lot of them. But we don't have that kind of world. We're profit driven.'

'That thought, of them profiting from your illness, is a tough one – I nearly said a hard pill to swallow.'

'It is, that's exactly what it is. But anyway, what was I saying, yes, I've changed a lot over the years and learned a lot. I see a world gone crazy, you know, a world gone crazy and I fear for the future.'

'So having MS has given you an opportunity to see life differently, and an effect of that is to fear for the future?'

Pauline stopped talking. She knew she was talking about things that, yes, they were important to her, but she was avoiding facing her own personal crisis. She'd managed to spend most of the session avoiding it, yet again, and she had to at least say something.

Jim has allowed Pauline the freedom to move through what is present for her. She has reconnected with her sense of what she needs to talk about and her feeling that she has been denying and avoiding it. Letting out some of her anger in the last few sentences has perhaps helped her regain perspective. Now, when the issue of her mobility is discussed, it is in response to her introducing it as it feels timely for her, and not as a result of the counsellor introducing it which could be at a time when something else is more present and pressing for the client. We deny things because they make us uncomfortable. Perhaps something from what has occurred in their dialogue has left Pauline more able to risk talking about her major issue. It might be Jim's openness about getting it wrong earlier, or his willingness to listen and take seriously thoughts and feelings that are important to her, or something else that emerged for Pauline within the experience of the counselling relationship.

'I'm avoiding here. I'm avoiding talking about whether or not I should start using a damned wheelchair.' She shook her head. 'I don't want to, I really don't want

to. I'm afraid that once I start I'll never get out of it, I'll weaken my leg muscles even more and that'll be that. I can't let that happen, I can't, but, oh I don't know. Diana thinks I should give it serious thought. I understand why. She has to lift me some days, and it's not good for her. But, oh God, I've spent the last 25 years trying to stop this happening, and now, now, now it's staring me in the face.'
'Yeah, staring you in the face, the one thing you've battled against for so long.'

Jim probably should have focused on the 'now, now, now . . .', this being Pauline's current issue, the fact that she is faced with the prospect of the wheelchair now. By so doing he would have perhaps conveyed to her a sense or feeling of affirmation that he has heard what lies at the heart of her struggle, facing the fact that it is happening *now*.

'And I don't know what to do, I really don't.'
'What to do, what to do?'
Pauline sat in silence and shook her head slightly. She had lowered her head and was looking down. The thought of a wheelchair – she really didn't want to, but she knew that it might make it easier, but at what cost? What would the cost be to her mobility, her legs, her muscles, her strength? Even the neurologist had mentioned it as being something to seriously consider but she wasn't going to tell her what to do.
'I don't know. I guess it'll have to happen one day, but I'm afraid of what effect it'll have on my legs, on the strength that I have. The thought of not walking.'
'So it's more the fear of the effect on your legs and the thought of not walking more than a fear of being in a wheelchair? Am I understanding you right, Pauline?'
'I've been in a chair, had to briefly, but I knew I'd get out of it. But this is different.'
'Yeah, now you don't know if you'll get out of it.'
'It's a battle, Jim. Every day is a battle. Throughout my life I've been forced to accept things that I can't do any more. It's never been easy, and I've always struggled on as long as I could. Working, driving, gardening – which I can't do because of the bending over – I've been forced to give up so much. Even this chair, you know, it's got a spring in it to help me up. I had to admit to needing it, but I know it's not an ordinary chair and since using this chair here it's made it more difficult to go anywhere where there are ordinary chairs. I can't sit on anything too low. And higher chairs don't often have arms to push up on. And I know I've lost strength since having this chair, and yet I know I need it. And I can see the same thing happening with a wheelchair.'
'That you'll lose strength and not be able to walk much, if at all.'
'It's the "if at all", Jim, that's what scares me. The thought of resigning myself to that fate.'
'Resigning yourself to not walking again.' How the hell do you make that decision, Jim thought to himself, and realised he hadn't got a clue. 'That's the terrifying thing.'

Pauline stared into space for a few moments. Being stuck in a wheelchair, she couldn't, not yet, she had to keep going somehow. But she was becoming more and more of a burden on Diana, and she had told her that, but Diana was always so good and understanding and always said it didn't matter. But it did, she knew it did. She knew it did. 'I don't know, Jim, I really don't. I'm not sure that I can make a decision. I guess I will do. I suppose in a way I am making the decision not to until the time comes when I feel ready to accept my fate. But I'm not making that choice now, I'm not there. But I guess I'm close, too bloody close for comfort.'

'So your sense is that because you haven't yet said "yes" to the wheelchair you are actually saying "no", but that it feels you are close to the day when you have to say "yes"?'

'It's getting close, I know it is, but I don't want to accept it. Not yet. I want to put it off a while longer, I really do. But, I don't know, I just don't know.'

There was so much tension present in the room. It was palpable. 'Close but not yet, but you just don't know. It's such a tense time; it feels tense to me and I'm not faced with the decision.'

'I hope you never are, Jim, I wouldn't wish this on anyone.'

'I appreciate that.' He nodded. 'I appreciate that.'

Pauline lapsed into silence again, not sure what else to say, and feeling that she knew at some level the inevitability of it all, and yet, not just yet, please, not just yet. But how much longer could she put it off? She didn't know. She was aware that talking to Jim this week had made her somehow more aware of the inevitability of it. It wasn't that they had really talked much about it, and she kind of knew it was out there waiting to happen to her, but somehow she was feeling more in touch with an acceptance of that inevitability. But not yet, not now. She was aware of feeling extremely tired once again, her eyes felt heavy and gritty and she felt she needed to end the session. She was feeling uncomfortable as well, and she needed to move around a bit in her chair, and wanted to walk about as well. Yes, she needed to get up and walk. But she decided to wait until after Jim had gone. She needed to prove it to herself.

'Jim, this session has really taken it out of me; can we leave it at that? It's been helpful. Yes, I think I am getting more accepting of the inevitability of being in a wheelchair. But not yet.'

Jim wasn't sure if she meant end the session or end the counselling. He voiced his uncertainty. 'You want to end this session, yeah. It has been heavy going, for both of us. I really do – I'm going to say something stupid I think – but I do admire you for letting me into your despair. It can't be easy. I just want to acknowledge that.'

'Not easy, but necessary, but you are easy to talk to and you do listen. And I appreciate that.'

The session drew to a close. They would meet again next week at the same time.

As Jim got back to his car he realised how tired he was himself after that session. He had been really concentrating and it had been so intense, so much feeling. Yes, he felt very affected, very touched by Pauline's despair and her struggle to remain able to walk. He could appreciate why she didn't want to accept a wheelchair and risk losing her own, natural mobility, and yet he could appreciate that there could be advantages too. But he wasn't there to give advice or his own opinion. She was getting that from others. He was there to offer her the non-directive space to explore her own feelings and thoughts and to discover for herself what she felt she wanted to do, what was acceptable to her.

Jim saw his supervisor twice a month, once to focus on his supervision work, and once on his counselling work. He was due to see him the next day for his supervision work, but he felt he wanted to talk about Pauline. He felt quite loaded up with reactions to her plight and felt he needed time to sift through them before he next saw her. He sometimes altered the content of the supervision sessions depending on what was most pressing. He felt he needed to do this to prepare himself for his next session with Pauline, both for her benefit and for his own well-being.

Points for discussion

- How are you left feeling towards Pauline? How might those feelings affect your offering of the core conditions to this client?
- What would you find challenging about seeing a client at their home for counselling?
- Evaluate the quality and the effectiveness of Jim's empathy.
- What do you feel are Jim's strengths and weaknesses as a counsellor?
- Do you feel it is acceptable to end a session early if a client is tiring and, if so, why from the standpoint of person-centred working?
- Contrast your own reaction to the two counselling sessions.
- Write notes for these sessions.

Learning Resources
Centre

CHAPTER 6

Supervision session 1: feeling powerless

David had been supervising Jim for a few months now; they were still building their supervisory relationship. David had grown to appreciate over those months the sincerity of Jim's practice. He really cared about his clients and, while he believed that this was an attitude necessary for effective therapy, there was something about Jim that seemed to take it a stage further. The warmth and respect that Jim reflected in the way he talked about his clients was inspiring and made it a joy for him to offer Jim supervision.

David didn't actually like thinking about what he offered in terms of it being 'supervision'; he didn't feel the term really reflected the quality and relational emphasis that good supervision required. He always found his supervision work touched him deeply. And he saw it as a very definite responsibility. Counsellors were working with clients, seeking to offer them authentic, therapeutic relationship. Yet he knew how the dynamics of the counsellor–client relationship could trigger all kinds of reactions in the counsellor which were not likely to be therapeutically valuable – indeed, which could damage the client. Yet he was left having to rely on what his supervisors wanted to raise, and even that meant that a certain screening could take place, and not necessarily consciously. Significant moments could simply be missed by the counsellor and, if not raised in supervision, could be missed again.

Yet in spite of this, David always felt that if he could get the supervisory relationship with his clients 'right', the actual material that needed addressing would emerge. If his relationship with his supervisees was such that it characterised the attitudinal qualities of the person-centred approach – congruence, empathy, unconditional positive regard – then what was present within the supervisee that was an expression of incongruence could, and would, begin to stand out. Often David found himself aware that there was something unexpressed that somehow felt important but he couldn't quite define exactly what it was. Invariably, when he trusted this inner prompting and voiced his concern, it led the supervisee into an area of themselves that proved to be significant for the work being done with the client.

Working with relationship – therapeutic relationship – David realised long ago was as much of an art as a science, and perhaps more so. The art of human relationship or relatedness. And what he had recognised was that for him to be genuinely sensitive to emerging incongruence within his supervisee, he needed to be sure that he was congruent, that his self-awareness was an accurate experience of his own process, and that he wasn't bringing his own 'conditions of worth' and 'introjects' into the supervisory relationship or, if he did, that he could identify them, own them, and put them to one side to be processed within his own supervision.

It was nearly time – Jim was a good time-keeper – so he took a moment to be aware of the flow of his own experiencing. The bell sounded and David got up to let Jim in.

David offered Jim a tea or coffee, as he always did to his supervisees, but Jim said no, he had not long had a drink. He settled into the supervision session. Jim highlighted that while he knew this session was for his own supervisory work, he wanted to check in with a new client who was very present for him. He said he would spend more time at the next supervision session, but wanted maybe ten minutes to acknowledge his own process in relationship with this client. David agreed and Jim began talking about his two sessions with Pauline. He gave an overview of the situation, of seeing her at home, of her relationship with Diana. And of her struggle to address her issue around whether or not to accept at this time the need to use a wheelchair.

David listened, not saying much, simply an occasional acknowledgement of what Jim had said. Finally Jim finished his overview. David was very aware that he had quite a clear picture of Pauline and her bungalow, all sound and tangible stuff, but he was acutely aware that he had little sense of Jim's reactions. Jim had presented Pauline in his usual sensitive and respectful way, but what was Jim feeling, how was he experiencing being with her, what impact was she having on the quality and nature of his empathy and his ability to maintain congruence? He did not doubt the presence of unconditional positive regard.

'I've got a really clear image of Pauline, Jim, and I am aware of not having much of a sense of how she is affecting you. I sensed your warmth, but it was all very factual and I'm aware that that isn't always your style. So I guess I'm wanting to flag up my wanting to have more of a sense of you in the relationship.'

David communicates that he has heard Jim's factual account, but he is not feeling connected to Jim, to what is happening within him. He makes this visible, owning his sense of what he feels he wants to hear, of what seems missing. The supervisor is inviting the counsellor to explore further, and at a deeper level, his relationship with his client.

Jim was slightly taken aback because he felt very much affected by Pauline, but maybe he wasn't communicating that. So that in itself was something to explore. 'I am feeling strongly affected, touched by her dilemma, but one of the feelings most present for me has been a sense of powerlessness. I mean in the sense that she's facing up to progressive disability with little hope of relief and real improvement, and it has left me feeling powerless in the face of this.'

'Mhmm, powerless to . . . ?'

Jim's response was in his head very quickly. 'To make it better, and I know that's not what counselling is about but it is my reaction to her struggle.'

'You really feel that powerlessness to help her in her struggle?'

Jim nodded and took a deep breath. It wasn't easy, he thought to himself, and he had a clear image of Pauline in that first session, in pain, struggling to move, and that cushion slipping. 'I feel for her, David, I really do feel for her. I'm so glad she has Diana and yet she's said how there are things she cannot talk to her about, or rather chooses not to. Shuts her out. She doesn't want to do that and, well, I guess I'm the opportunity for her to find another way.'

David nodded, noting to himself that that was a powerful effect to have on a client, but he didn't want to draw that conclusion for Jim. He'd rather Jim made that recognition for himself. He wanted Jim to evaluate his own influence on Pauline. 'Mhmm, maybe though the relationship she will feel able to talk in ways she hasn't been able to before. Yes, you're giving her opportunity.'

'I hope she takes it, I really do. She needs to talk it through and I need to be able to listen without giving her a direction or somehow encouraging her in any way.'

'I'm struck by a wonder as to whether you feel you might do this?'

'I don't know. I mean, I don't know what's best for her. I hear her dilemma and probably not knowing what's best is good; I can really help her to freely explore the issues, her feelings, her fears, her hopes, whatever is present. I hope I can do that and keep it open. I'm sure she needs that.'

'So is there anything in particular you need to be able to offer to facilitate this?' David was wanting to encourage Jim to explore this more, to help him be sure he could offer to Pauline what he sensed was important for her to ensure she could most effectively use the therapeutic relationship.

'I need to keep my empathy clear and accurate. I have to avoid opinions, and I may develop some as she explores it. I am sure I will, perhaps drawing in my own mind conclusions that may be different to hers.' Jim thought for a moment about that. As he heard himself speaking he realised that it wasn't something he had fully appreciated. 'That's a real problem, I know that. Of course I'm going to develop my own ideas, I can't avoid that, and I need to keep them to myself.' He paused, feeling quite clear on this. 'But what if Pauline asks a direct question? I can respond by acknowledging the importance of her decision and that maybe she feels she wants another opinion, but that sounds a bit naff and counsellor-speak to me. I want to be genuine, but I don't want to direct her. Shit. I'm not sure. What do I do? I don't know.'

'So if she asks you a direct question, wanting your opinion, you want to be authentic with her but you don't want to direct her. You don't want to come across in a naff kind of way.'

> It can be tempting to give an opinion, but it would step outside of the non-directive nature of counselling. The counselling relationship offers the client opportunity to move around their own inner world freely and without, hopefully, the therapist telling them what to do or what conclusion to draw. In this instance, David now goes on to clarify Jim's role, reminding him that the client can gain advice from outside the therapeutic relationship.

'No, I want to be helpful, but I want to help her make her own decision.'

'So, your role is clear, a place, a space, in which she can explore options, but not a place in which you give her options, or give opinions about her options. She gets those from outside your relationship and brings them into it, yes?'

Jim nodded. 'Yes, that makes sense, and she does have access to information. She's clued up about it. She's part of this local support group. I'm not sure what discussions she may have had with other people in a similar positions, I kind of sense that she hasn't.'

'So, you're not sure what she'll bring into the sessions in terms of information.'

'No, and I think in a way it's more about gut feeling and fear for her as much as anything. That's what she is bottling up, that makes it hard to talk about it. She is holding her fears down under pressure and is afraid of not being able to control them if she lets the pressure out.'

'And maybe she needs to let the pressure out before she can take the information on board. That's my view, I realise that, but sometimes we cannot really hear the information clearly and make a truly informed choice about something until we have processed our feelings.'

'And sometimes we simply act on feelings regardless of the information and the thinking!'

David smiled. 'Yes, true. But what is your sense of Pauline?'

'She's bottled up a lot of fear, she really does feel a lot hinges on her decision now, and I can't rush her, can't give her an answer. She's going to have to take her time and really contemplate this one until she is sure of what she wants to do.'

'And we can contemplate change for a long time, or sometimes very quickly.'

'Yes. And I know that. It's the "cycle of change", isn't it, that was devised to explain the process of making choices around addictions. Pre-contemplation of change followed by contemplation, preparation, action and hopefully maintenance. And relapse or lapse if the person is unable to sustain change.' [Prochaska and DiClemente, 1982]

'It's a good model and, yes, Pauline is contemplating change.'

Jim was aware that this angle on it was helping him. He knew you didn't try to get ahead of clients in contemplation, but you facilitated their exploration of the pros and cons. Yes, he could have that in mind as he worked with her, and that felt good. Having that framework in the back of his mind would, he felt, make a difference. He certainly felt a difference thinking about it now. He actually suddenly felt he had something to offer in the sense that he wasn't powerless. Well, he was to make Pauline better, but he could have a powerful effect on her if he could really facilitate her process of contemplating what she was going to do about the wheelchair. Would she make a change, or would she choose her current level of mobility for a bit longer? He didn't know, but he felt he could apply his person-centred attitudes and values to this way of looking at Pauline's dilemma, and bring person-centred working and the cycle of change model together. [Bryant-Jefferies, 2001]

The discussion moved on to other work that Jim was doing, but he was grateful for having spent the time talking about Pauline. He was now more able to acknowledge where his powerlessness rightly lay, and also where he felt he could be powerfully present within the therapeutic relationship.

Counselling session 3: 'accepting me' and 'anxious me'

The session had begun with Pauline commenting on how tired she was after the last session, that she had in fact fallen asleep and been woken by Diana coming in a little while later. However, she indicated that she was feeling more alert this week; she hadn't been in so much pain again and had been getting better nights' sleep. So she felt positive coming into the session and intended to focus more on what she really wanted to talk about, what to do about her mobility.

Jim had responded by acknowledging that he appreciated what Pauline wanted to focus on, and he continued, 'So, where do you want to begin?'

Pauline sat and pondered for a short while. Where did she want to begin? So many factors seemed to be around for her to consider, so many different opinions, arguments for and against. Where to begin? She felt a certain anxiety as she began to speak.

'It's the fear of what I might lose by admitting to myself that I need to use a wheelchair.'

'What you might lose . . .'

'Like I said before, the less I use my legs, the weaker they'll get and I'm not at all sure that will be a good idea. I need to keep them strong, at least to some degree. Otherwise, well . . .' She took a deep breath, '. . . otherwise I really will be crippled for life.'

'That's the fear, that admitting to needing a wheelchair now will leave you crippled for life.' Jim sought to empathically sum up what he had heard Pauline saying. He added, 'It's that fear of what you might lose . . .'

The power of empathy. The client is ready to talk about her anxiety and the person-centred counsellor keeps his responses fairly short and focused. Where empathy is leading into a deeper connection within the client, there can be a sense of the seriousness of the moment. The person-centred counsellor will be making a particular effort to stay focused on the client and what she is communicating to him.

Pauline could feel herself going silent and a knot developing in the pit of her sto-mach. She knew she had to keep going, somehow, had to keep herself on her legs. She wasn't old enough to retreat to a wheelchair. That's what it felt like, a retreat, giving up, she nearly found herself thinking in terms of running away – she shook her head slightly, stupid idea that. She wasn't capable of running anywhere, and she never would, ever again. That thought got to her. The knot had extended and she could feel tears welling up in her eyes. Silly old fool, she thought to herself, and hunted around for a tissue, eventually finding one and dabbing her eyes as tears began to trickle down her cheeks.

Jim kept his attention on Pauline. Fear, he thought to himself, fear of losing your ability to walk. As he sat there knowing that he could just get up without any thought and move wherever he wanted without any pain, he reminded himself how much he took it for granted. And here was Pauline: no movement was pain-free and facing the thought of losing her ability to walk.

Pauline took another deep breath and looked up at Jim. 'It's a bugger of a choice.'

Jim nodded. 'Yeah, a real bugger.'

'I feel so helpless sometimes and I hate it, I hate feeling reliant on Diana, hate it. If I didn't walk a little bit, well, I'd be more reliant, more of a burden. Can't do that. I just can't do that.'

'No, the thought of burdening Diana is too much, far too much. You can't do that.'

'And yet I know that one day I will have to resign myself to my fate. But has that time arrived. Has it? Part of me is saying yes, another part is saying no. And I just don't know what's for the best, for me, for Diana. I don't know.'

'Different parts of you with different views, and you're left between them, not knowing, just not knowing.' Jim sought to stay with Pauline, seeking to com-municate empathy for what she was saying, how she was describing what she was feeling.

'It's like one is saying, no, whatever you do, not that. Not that. Think about how you'd feel, how uncomfortable it would be. Sitting there, watching your legs waste away.' She closed her eyes. The image was too much for her, too vivid. The tears began to flow again, and she sobbed. It seemed to Jim that however much it sounded like a cliché, she was sobbing her heart out. He felt saddened for her, for the image that she was now facing.

'It's an awful thought, horrible to contemplate, so horrible to contemplate.' He spoke gently, letting Pauline know what he was sensing to be her feelings towards the image.

'It feels so awful that it's like it's beyond awful. And I don't have words for how it makes me feel. It's just . . . ughh, I can't bear it.' She had closed her eyes again and the sobbing continued.

Jim has been in a sense doubling up on his empathy by repeating himself: 'can't do that', 'just not knowing', 'so horrible to contemplate'. He may not be doing this wittingly, but it is likely to have a powerful effect, holding the client that little while longer each time on what she has said, what she is feeling. It slows the dialogue down, introducing more space for the client to acknowledge what is present for her. This style is not a technique. If it was deliberately applied to produce an effect it would not be person-centred working, because it would immediately flow from an agenda, a goal, an intention to make the client feel or experience something which, presumably, the counsellor thinks they need to feel. But where it is a spontaneous response to the depth and strength of the feelings that the client is conveying, then it is going to be an empathic response emerging out of the counsellor's experience of what the client is communicating, and therefore a valid person-centred response.

Jim got up, squatted down closer to Pauline and leaned across to touch her arm. He felt he had to reach out in some way, he guessed as much for himself as perhaps for Pauline. But he couldn't sit just observing her distress. It felt invasive, voyeuristic almost. He needed to make some kind of human response and he had heard and appreciated what Pauline had said about not having the words. So he was making a non-verbal communication.

Pauline felt his touch. It was gentle; she guessed he was hesitant in case it caused her pain. In fact it tickled slightly and her arm twitched in response.

Jim felt the movement and took it to be a pulling away so he withdrew his hand.

'It tickled, that's all. I appreciate your reaching out. People often seem frightened to touch me in case they cause me discomfort.'

'That was my concern, but I wanted to take that risk. I wanted to reach out to you and it felt like it needed to be something other than words.' He touched her forearm again but with a little more pressure this time. Pauline took another deep breath. It did feel somehow reassuring, that contact. But she wasn't really thinking very much. She was just sitting, being with a lot of feelings that were welling up inside her, among them the fear she had already mentioned, but increasingly a kind of wobbliness that left her feeling sort of shaky, but on the inside. And she felt hot. She took another deep breath and let it out slowly. 'What am I going to do, Jim? I'm in a right old mess here, aren't I? I can't stay like this. I'm beginning to wonder if it's worse simply not making a decision. All that does is leave me worrying about it even more.'

Jim nodded. 'Yeah, I can understand that, how it must leave you with the same fears and anxieties. It's like you have to make a decision.'

As she heard Jim's response the realisation dawned on her – well, she kind of knew it but hadn't really engaged with the thought – that actually it wasn't really a decision about should she admit to needing a wheelchair or not. It was not a case of if, but when, when would she succumb to wheels. When. Not if. She nodded slightly. She voiced her thoughts. 'It's no longer a matter of "if" I should use a wheelchair, it's become "when". It's out there, waiting for me, isn't it, and I'm going to have to accept it.'

'That's how it feels, it's when not if, and it's waiting for you, there's inevitability.'

'I knew that, I mean, I sort of knew it, like, well, you know it'll happen but always further ahead, when you're a lot older. But look at me, 53, that's all, I should be looking forward to my second half of life, to retirement.' She shook her head. 'Well, I am retired, and what have I got to look forward to?'

'What have you got to look forward to?'

'A lot of pain, more physical complication – bowel and bladder problems, and maybe problems with my eyes as well, and some people it affects their ability to swallow too. Finding I can do less and less with a body that's getting messed up more and more.'

'Pain, more complications, and doing less and less.' Jim had noticed a padded stool over by the table on the other side of the room. 'I'd like to go and get that stool and sit on it. Is that OK? I kind of feel a bit distant sitting over there on the settee. But is that OK with you?'

'Sure. Please, get it. But will you be comfortable?'

Will *I* be comfortable, Jim thought! 'Yes, I'm sure I'll be OK, and if not, I'll move. That OK?'

'Sure.'

Jim went over and got the stool. It was nicely padded. He brought it back and set it down about midway between the settee and where Pauline was sitting. It felt close enough to reach out to her, but distant enough so as not to be in her space – at least, that's how he felt but he checked it out. 'Is that OK – not too close?'

Pauline felt OK about where Jim was now sitting. She realised she'd have been uneasy if he'd suggested this in the first session, but already she was feeling more comfortable with him. 'That's fine.'

'OK. So where were we? Yes, feeling that you only had pain and being able to do less and less in the future.'

Pauline was silent. Yes, that's how it was. And she was already finding that on some days the walls kind of closed in, or rather, the world outside seemed to become more distant, less accessible, more uneasy to think about.

'I find it hard to go out some days, I've noticed in the last few weeks even that I find reasons to stay in. Seems such a struggle and when you're in pain, the noise, the bustle, everything can get too much. I feel like I just want a quiet life. And yet I know that I don't. My mind is active, I want to be involved in things, but my bloody legs won't let me!'

Jim felt the exasperation in Pauline's voice. But to say something about how exasperated he felt she was somehow sounded all wrong; at least, the word was too long.

'Pisses you off, huh, good and proper.'

> Jim has chosen to express his empathic sense of what Pauline experiencing rather than the words she has used, recognising that what she is actually experiencing is probably feeling fed up and pissed off by the whole experience.

Pauline had to smile. Yeah, that summed it up, wasn't quite what she'd expected Jim to say, but yeah, she was pissed off. It felt good, somehow, hearing him say that, kind of helped her to acknowledge that, yeah, that's how it was. 'Yeah, pissed off, fucking pissed off.' Her lips tightened. 'Dammit, this is going nowhere. I know what I'm facing and I can't make the decision – I don't want to make it, you know? It's ...' she closed her eyes, 'it's just too terrifying.' She felt a wave of panic hit her and she struggled to regain her composure. 'The thought of never walking again, though, I mean, it's the thin end of a wedge. Once I start to use a wheelchair regularly, that's it. It'll be hard to make myself walk, to try and keep my mobility.'

'That's what you sense will happen, you'll find yourself using the wheelchair more and spend less and less time using your legs.'

'Of course I will. Of course I will.' Pauline lapsed back into silence. She was thinking about whether there might be a compromise. The thought of being stuck in a wheelchair – that was how it felt – was too much. She couldn't make a decision that faced her with that prospect, not yet, not at her age. But could she maybe just use it occasionally? Could she? Would she? She didn't know. She suspected not, but could it be there for the bad days? Yet she knew she needed to use her leg muscles pretty regularly to keep their strength and maintain some of her mobility. She had started doing some leg exercises on better days, to try and keep some muscle tone.

Jim was hearing Pauline saying how she was terrified, and believed that she would just use a wheelchair more and more. And yet something within was nagging at him. It didn't have to be like that. He saw people on different kinds of motorised chairs and some of them were very different-looking to wheelchairs. But that was easy for him to think. He wasn't the one facing it. He knew instinctively that to say anything that encouraged a compromise or a different view to the one Pauline had would be a stepping out of role. Pauline had said right at the start – well, early on in that first session, from what he could recall – that she didn't want suggestions or opinions. She wanted space to reach her own decision. And however difficult it is to sit with Pauline's process, it's nothing compared to what Pauline herself is feeling.

He didn't say anything. In truth, he wasn't too sure what to say. The silence had continued long enough for it to feel odd to suddenly respond to what Pauline had last said. He didn't want to voice his own reflection and risk taking Pauline away from her own focus. So he stayed silent, keeping his attention on Pauline and being open to the feelings that were present for him towards her. He really did care about her, and he really did appreciate the magnitude of her decision. He voiced it. 'The more I sit with you and listen to you, the more I appreciate the magnitude of your dilemma, Pauline, of the decision you are faced with. I can't tell you what to do, I don't know what's right for you, what you need to do. But I want to help you find a way through all of this, however long it takes and whatever the outcome.' He was looking at Pauline, who had lifted her head and was looking back into his eyes. It felt a profound moment.

Pauline felt a strange quiet, a kind of momentary connectedness and yet it felt like forever. For Jim, there was a calmness. Pauline sensed the genuineness in what Jim had just said. It was an expression of himself, not a reflection and a response to something she had said. And it felt good. It felt like he had become more present. He already was present, she knew that, but now she kind of felt it as well. No, she'd felt it before, but it was like a deeper, more present kind of feeling. They maintained the eye contact.

Jim was determined not to break the connection. He trusted these moments. They seemed to involve a reaching out, but more than that. A meeting of two people, perhaps their minds, maybe their feelings, sometimes both. Two people making a person-to-person connection in an atmosphere of genuine and greater openness than what was usually present between people. In his view this kind of connection was one of the most powerful and healing experiences in the world. He held his eye contact and the feelings of positive regard that were present within him towards Pauline.

Jim had broken the silence by offering his own experience, quietly and sincerely. It has led to a moment of deepening connection. His decision to break the silence is something that cannot be easily evaluated. It is simply one of those moments in therapy when the counsellor knows there is something present for them that has to be communicated to the client. The therapeutic value can only be measured by the impact it has on the client and the effect it has on the relationship in the moments that follow. These moments of what can seem inspired intervention seem to emerge from a deep place within the counsellor and are often coloured by a sense of knowing the rightness in speaking. There is a profound connection between the therapist and the client.

However, this should not be regarded as an excuse for a counsellor to say anything that they feel, definitely not that. It is deeper, more profound, more ... It's hard to put into words, but you know these moments when you have experienced them, either as a counsellor or as a client. They will be therapeutically helpful, although the precise outcome cannot be known in advance. Both client and counsellor will make of them whatever meaning they choose to attach to the experience.

Pauline felt Jim's warmth and sincerity. There was a gentleness present and she had noted this before. He seemed to offer a kind of quiet reassurance. He didn't seem flustered at all, but he seemed to be able to be quite calm, and yet it wasn't as though he disappeared in the calm. He remained very present. She felt good that she had chosen him to be her counsellor. She'd spoken to someone else, but she hadn't really seemed right. That had surprised her. She thought she would have gone for a female counsellor. But she hadn't.

She was struck by the thought that actually what was most helpful was Jim's presence rather than what he said. It was the sense that he was listening and keeping his attention focused on her. Yes, it was his presence that was important, a kind and calm presence that somehow seemed to offer a kind of strength to face things. And yet rationally she knew that didn't make sense. She'd only had less than three hours with him, and yet time didn't seem to matter. She felt a connection, she felt that he was . . . she just kept coming back to the same word, it was something about his presence. She took a deep breath.

'I seem to draw strength from you, at least, I feel somehow stronger.'

'Something about me gives you strength?'

'Not sure if you're giving it or I'm taking it, or maybe it's helping me to connect with myself, but I do get strength from this. It's not that it makes it better or even easier, but I seem to feel able to face things.'

Jim felt appreciation for what Pauline had said. He was glad he was having that effect and he voiced it. 'I'm pleased that what I am offering is helping in this way, Pauline. I'm not sure that counselling makes things easier; I think it can make it harder because it can enable people to become more self-aware and that may mean being more aware of difficult areas.' Jim was aware that he had strayed into talking about the process of counselling rather than specifically staying with Pauline, so he added, 'But it leaves you feeling more able to face things.'

'Somehow, yes. I feel like I know that I have to accept the wheelchair. It's like, deep down, really deep down, I know it.'

'Really deep down you know it . . .'

'But I don't want to accept it. Another part of me is kind of trying to keep me away from what kind of feels like resigning myself to my fate.'

'Mhmm, that sounds pretty clear to me, Pauline, one deeper part knowing the inevitability and accepting it, but another part trying to push it aside.' As he said the last bit he made a pushing aside movement with his hands.

'More of a pushing down.' Pauline lifted her hands and pushed down in front of her.

'Like you're trying to bury it?' Jim was glad he had made the arm movement – it had perhaps opened up the possibility of clearer understanding.

'Something like that. It doesn't feel to the side, it feels deeper, underneath. It's like there's this part of me saying, "You know it's gonna happen, might as well get used to it, learn to make the best of it", but the other part doesn't want to hear that.'

Jim nodded. 'Two parts, one conveying a knowing that it is inevitable and you'd better get used to it, make the best of it, and another part I guess terrified of it and trying to push the thoughts back down, trying to get them out of the way.'

'Yes, yes, that's true. The terror is very much in the part that doesn't want to know. The other part of me feels kind of accepting of it all. Yes, that's weird. But the terror can overwhelm me and it does.'

'The terror overwhelms and, what, stops you hearing that more accepting part of yourself?'

'Stops me, yes . . .' Pauline was thinking about all of this. Yes, there was a part of her that did accept it but it was hard to really tune into. And yet somehow, just now, it had felt more present. 'That deeper part was feeling more present just now, and yet already I can feel myself experiencing anxiety and it's making it kind of fade.'

'Mhmm. Fades as you experience more anxiety?'

Pauline shook her head. 'I can see them clearly, you know, but it's like one gets stronger and the other gets weaker?'

'Mhmm, and the accepting part weakens as you feel more anxious.'

'The accepting part, it's like . . .' Pauline was trying to get a feel for what it was. She didn't want to feel the anxiety; it was uncomfortable. The accepting part seemed more at ease, somehow. 'It's like, yes, a part of me that, well, takes things in its stride.'

'OK, so there is a deep, accepting part of you that takes things in its stride.'

'And that's been very much me, you know, finding ways to cope, making the best out of things. But the thought of the wheelchair, that just washes it away.'

'Washes it away, leaving you . . . ?'

'Sort of – this'll sound weird – kind of back in the me that is getting by as things are. It's like part of me just doesn't want to know and the anxiety puts up a barrier and I think can leave me, temporarily at least, not thinking about the wheelchair, but it doesn't last.'

'I need to check out that I'm hearing you as you want me to understand what you are saying. The part of you that is anxious about accepting a wheelchair kind of gives you temporary relief from worrying about it, but then it comes back.'

Pauline listened and was thinking about it. 'And that sounds like a contradiction and yet somehow that's what it feels like. I get stuck in that part of me that doesn't want to know and I get really anxious, terrified, make a kind of commitment to not let it happen and just carry on as I am. That makes me feel a little more at ease, knowing that I'm not going to let it happen. But it doesn't last. It's like the two parts of me are constantly struggling with each other, except, no . . . That's not right. It's only the anxious me that's struggling. Struggling to keep the accepting me at bay. The accepting me is much more . . . well, accepting. Stupid thing to say!'

'That's how it feels, though, there is, and I use your words, an "anxious me" and an "accepting me" – "anxious me" is struggling to keep "accepting me" at a distance.'

Pauline nodded. 'That's how it is.'

It seemed to Jim that Pauline was identifying what have become known as 'configurations within self' (Mearns, 1999; Mearns and Thorne, 2000) – constellations of feelings, thoughts and behaviours that have developed within the structure of self. One part accepts the reality and inevitability of the wheelchair, and is maybe resigned to it. That part is probably fed up with the struggle and just wants some ease from it all. Yet over the years Pauline has developed an 'anxious me' in relation to losing her mobility, her independence. This part cannot survive if the acceptance is allowed to dominate and govern Pauline's behaviour. So 'anxious me' seeks to keep in control, emerging to push the acceptance aside through her anxiety state. Both are equally valid aspects of Pauline's structure of self, requiring warm acceptance by the counsellor. Both have voices; both want to be heard.

'Mhmm.' Jim waited, allowing Pauline to be with her thoughts and her processing of what she was recognising in her self. It felt crucially important and he didn't want to introduce anything external to her process. Pauline was exploring the landscape of her inner world. She didn't need his footprints all over it, or him effectively telling her what she was seeing. Rather let her look around and, when she feels ready, tell me in her own words what she sees, what she is experiencing. He maintained his feeling of positive regard and waited, attentively.

As she thought about the part of her that seemed accepting of her situation she could actually feel anxiety rising within her. It really felt like her 'anxious me' did not want to let any acceptance emerge. Strange business, she thought, sitting here thinking like this. But she could feel the anxiety, it was very present. 'It's all leaving me feeling very anxious, that part of me seems to rise up at the thought of accepting that I need to use a wheelchair.' As she said it she could feel tension inside her body, particularly in her chest. Yet she felt somehow there was something irrational about it, like it just would not let her hardly think about the possibility of using a wheelchair. 'Every time I try to think about it, wham, in comes the anxiety, and it's irrational, it's a pure reaction, no thoughts in my head at all about what I am anxious about. Seems like I am more anxious about the possibility that I might make the decision to have a wheelchair. But I can't get near to it at the moment, the anxiety keeps rising up.'

'It just keeps breaking through and creating a kind of barrier, keeping the accepting part of you away.'

Pauline was amazed at what was happening, what she was experiencing. She had never experienced anything quite like it before. She could feel herself moving into the anxiety, and the worry, and the thoughts about losing her mobility, the little strength she had left in her legs. 'I can't go into a wheelchair, I can't. I've too much to lose. It might be an awful mistake. I mean, I can't risk losing my strength. I really can't.' Her heart was pounding, really thumping. And she was aware that her chest had tightened. She swallowed and tried to slow down her breathing, trying to take slow, deep breaths. She could feel herself going cold and yet she felt damp, a kind of cold sweat. Her arms felt heavy.

'You really can't go into a wheelchair, so much to risk losing. It's leaving you incredibly anxious.' Jim wanted to convey his understanding of what Pauline was saying as well as what he sensed was present judging by her tone of voice, which seemed very anxious, verging on the panicky. He was wondering whether Pauline might experience a panic attack. She looked very frightened, and it had come on quite suddenly. She had really connected with something within herself and it was powerful.

'No, I have to keep my independence, I have to hang on to some power, I have to. I can't give in, mustn't give in, must never give in.'

Jim was struck by the word 'never'. That was unrealistic (from his frame of reference), but so often, and understandably, any retreat in the face of progressive disability was felt to be an act of giving in. He knew that Pauline, if she chose to accept her need for a wheelchair now or in the near future, wouldn't have given in. It would be out of necessity. The thought crossed his mind that there would probably be some advantages, but he knew that was his thinking and it wasn't for him to introduce that into Pauline's current frame of reference. He conveyed back to her the significant words in what she had said. 'Independence, power, must never give in, never give in.'

'No.' As she spoke Pauline found herself feeling different. Hearing Jim seemed to have caused something to change. 'I can't give in. I have to keep going.' Yet she felt somehow that her heart wasn't really in what she was saying. She was tired of keeping going, that was the truth of it. She wanted a break; she wanted it a bit easier. Would she get that with a wheelchair, would she? She just didn't know. Again her heart was thumping. She couldn't seem to get away from the feelings of unease. She knew that at this present moment in time she could not make a decision other than to carry on, seeking to do the best she could. 'I can't make the decision to go for a wheelchair, Jim, I know I can't. I'm not there. But I'm beginning to recognise that one day I will be, and, well, maybe that will be sooner, maybe later, I don't know. Maybe something will leave me making that decision quicker than I think. But I'm not there now, not today. It just leaves me too anxious to really think clearly.'

Jim nodded. 'Yes, the anxiety just overwhelms you.'

'Am I being silly? Should I be really, seriously contemplating a wheelchair?'

Jim's ears pricked up at the word 'contemplating'. Part of the 'cycle of change', he realised he was thinking to himself. 'Contemplating something to make a decision about can take a long time.'

'I know, maybe a lifetime.'

'Maybe. I guess we make decisions when, for whatever reason, the time feels right for us. Maybe you just don't feel the time is right for you yet to make a decision to start to use a wheelchair.'

'Maybe.' Pauline was feeling herself coming over tired again, and she was aware that the session hadn't run its time. Her eyes felt suddenly heavy once again. 'I'm struggling again. It just comes over me.' She yawned. 'Sorry.'

'That's OK, it's been an intense time for you again. Must take it out of you, particularly when you are concentrating on difficult feelings.' Jim could see Pauline was struggling. He offered to end the session and give her time to recover a bit. Pauline agreed to this and they drew the session to a close.

> The tiredness might be a genuine reaction to the intensity of the session; however, it could be an element within Pauline using tiredness to block what is occurring in terms of the conclusion she is reaching. Pauline is saying that she may not be ready now to make the decision about the wheelchair, but maybe one day in the future she will be. That is a clear and valid assessment. It is again threatening, though, to that part of her that is saying 'never' give in. Obtusely, the 'never give in' part could be invoking tiredness to stop the process.

Jim offered shorter sessions in case Pauline felt that might be more manageable, but she declined. 'No, I want to give myself the opportunity of the full session. It's important to me. What happened today has given me a lot to think about. I've experienced myself in a new way, feeling quite distinct parts to myself. I'd never really seen myself quite like that, not so distinctly. I need to think about all of this, take it all in.'

The session ended. Jim left, feeling tired himself. He realised how much he had been concentrating on Pauline, particularly during her silences. He felt stiff and was stretching his back as he went to open the car door. Made him realise once again how grateful he was to be able to stand here and stretch himself like this. He hadn't given it a moment's thought, walking down the path. But for Pauline, for her to walk that path each step would be painful and, on bad days, impossible to make. He was glad he was working with her. It was affecting his own perspective on life and on himself. He had noted how, since working with Pauline, he was more conscious of walking, of his movement, and he had caught himself on more than one occasion taking delight in the feeling of movement in his legs and arms. He sat for a moment before starting the car engine. 'Yes, I'm lucky,' he spoke out aloud. He hadn't noticed the woman walking past his car window with her dog as he spoke. She gave him a funny look and kept walking. He smiled. Oh well, it was how he felt. He knew that he was appreciating his own health and well-being. He knew that at some level he couldn't take it for granted any more. In a way he saw this as a gift from Pauline and he was grateful for that.

Counselling session 4: a change of attitude and Pauline's body mourns

Jim was spending a few moments in his car before the session. He had arrived a little early. He wanted to feel centred and open to the flow of experiencing within him in preparation for the session. He closed his eyes and allowed himself to be with what was present. His thoughts went to Pauline and the last session. He felt uncertain as to what decision Pauline was going to reach. He was so aware of the two aspects of herself that she had identified last week, and how strong and controlling her anxiety could be. Yet his sense was that her accepting part of the reality or at least the inevitability of a wheelchair was probably something that was developing and at some point might assume a power of its own equal to that of her anxiety. He put his speculation aside and took a couple of deep breaths before getting out of his car.

Jim pressed the buzzer and Diana came to the door. 'Hi, come on through. Pauline's in the lounge.'

'Thanks.' Jim walked through, glad that Diana hadn't sought to engage in further conversation. He felt that he needed to keep his focus with Pauline and it seemed that Diana respected that.

'Hi, Jim, sit down.'

'Thanks.' He noticed that the seat he had used last week had already been moved over to Pauline's side of the lounge, so he sat there. 'I see you've moved this over. Thanks for that. I don't know about you, but it felt a bit distant sitting over there on the settee.'

'Yes, and I did appreciate your presence last week; it felt very important. That session really drained me again, and I want to look at that today. I've been thinking about things a lot, and trying to analyse my anxiety and my acceptance of my fate.'

'Mhmm.' Jim said nothing more; clearly Pauline had things to say and he let her continue, just responding minimally to affirm his attention.

'Well, it seems to me that I need to work on that acceptance. I can't cope with the anxiety, it doesn't do me any good. Sitting here worrying about things. It takes over and it just gets in the way. I don't like it and I'm fed up with it.'

To Jim she sounded quite flat – a real sense of having had enough. 'Yes, had enough of the anxiety taking over, and the worrying.'

A crucial feature of person-centred working is acceptance of the client as they are in the session. They may be where they left off the previous week, but more likely different experiences will have moved them to another place, or they will have a different view of their situation. The therapist has to be open to the client as they are and put aside their memory of how they were. A lot can change in a week. The client may want to communicate what is present and real for them now, and the counsellor needs to be open, attentive and responsive to this. Even though the person-centred approach is not in the business of setting clients 'homework', nevertheless work is done 'at home' during the week, processes continue, and much time can be spent reflecting on the content or the implications of the previous session. As with Pauline, greater self-insight can emerge, leaving her clearer about her internal process and the areas within herself that she needs to address.

Pauline continued. 'I know that deep down I really do accept it, I really do, but then there's another part of me that won't allow me to accept it. And that struggle between them, it tires me out. And I'm tired of the struggle. I'm tired of a lot of things, actually.' She paused before continuing, 'Tired of the illness, of the pain, of dragging myself around. It's not always there. I mean, I have good days and, yes, I really don't dwell on things so much then and I can enjoy things, you know, and laugh and have a joke. But that's so difficult on the bad days.'

'Yeah, the bad days stop you laughing, joking, feeling in touch with a sense of enjoyment. You're tired of it all.'

'And there's part of me that thinks that accepting a wheelchair is giving up, and I can't give up. And yet I also know that it could be a positive choice, perhaps. I don't know. My thinking's been challenged a bit this week. I was feeling good and went to an MS group meeting, and got chatting to a new lady there, hadn't seen her before, and she had one of these motorised ... not exactly a buggy, more of a scootery kind of thing, you know? Not the typical wheelchair, much more stylish, and solid. And, well, we got chatting and I said about how I was struggling to accept my fate. Anyway, she told me about her experience, and how she had experienced similar feelings, and really didn't want to accept her fate either, but she had been persuaded to give it a go, if only as a temporary measure, or on bad days, but to give herself a bit more freedom to get about. Anyway, funny that, I never really saw it as something giving freedom, always thinking about how limiting it would be because I'd not be using my legs.' She paused, still aware that she hadn't really taken that fully on board yet.

'Mhmm, so she saw it as liberating, you see it as being shackled? Is that too strong a contrast?' Jim was sensing extremes; it was something about the way Pauline had spoken, and the degree of almost surprise in her voice when she had spoken about what the lady had said about giving freedom. But maybe his use of language had gone a bit too far.

Pauline thought about that. Liberated and shackled, was that how it was? Shackled sounded really extreme, unable to move, but yes, that was how she saw a wheelchair. It would leave her unable to really move much on her legs, or that was her fear. 'That really sharpens it up, what you just said. Really does make you think.'

'Mhmm, makes you think. Liberation or being shackled.' Jim sought to keep with Pauline, stay with her in her focus as she experienced her own reactions to this notion.

Pauline was still silent. She was very much in her own thoughts. That sense of fearing the effects of using a wheelchair was being challenged by what the lady had said – Isabel was her name – Isabel had really been so positive and enthusiastic. But she struggled to see herself in that motorised buggy. 'I just can't see myself in one of those motorised buggies. I can't imagine, somehow ...' She was thinking of how the world would look. She'd be stuck in the chair, probably. 'I'd feel limited. I mean, I can't walk too well, but at least I can sort of go where I want when I'm feeling good, except for steps that is, and a wheelchair wouldn't get me up them anyway.'

Jim noted that the fearful side of her had developed another argument against it – the sense of feeling limited. He voiced what he was understanding her to say. 'That sense of not being able to imagine what it would be like, and of feeling limited.'

'Always looking at the world from down here, that's the thought that has struck me, and that's weird, I mean, that doesn't really matter, but somehow that's important as well.'

'The notion of sitting and looking out on the world from a seated position, that's kind of important.'

'Somehow very important. It's hard to imagine, I mean, I have been in a wheelchair after operations and I do know what it is like, but that's in a different setting and for a different purpose. It's like you're there for a while. There's a purpose to using the chair. But to have to use one for everything . . .'

'Everything? I'm very struck by a sense of the all-or-nothing way that you see it, Pauline.' Jim wanted to be open about his own experience of listening to Pauline. This notion had been developing for some time, but it felt particularly present and persistent at this time.

Jim empathises with the nature of what is being said as much as with the content.

'That's sort of what Isabel was saying. She said that to begin with she only used it when she needed to use it, not all the time. She said it made life easier, that it had actually broadened her horizons somewhat as well. She could go out to places with her husband and take her other chair – she has two chairs, the one I saw her with, and more of a powered wheelchair that she uses when they travel distances. She doesn't use a manual wheelchair, her husband gets breathless easily and it would put too much of a strain on him. So she has this powered wheelchair which she literally drives into the back of the car – they've got a converted car to take it. She says that sometimes she'll get out of the chair and sit in the front of the car, she prefers that, and that her husband puts the chair in the back. But on bad days when she still wants to go out, she just drives it up a ramp and into the back of the car, and it's kind of clamped in and she has a special seat belt.' Pauline paused, before continuing. 'She says it's OK for journeys up to 30 or 40 miles, beyond that she much prefers to be in the front. Anyway, I've arranged to go round and have a look at their set-up on Friday. She just seemed such a positive, outgoing lady, and I just felt, yes, what she's saying makes sense. She also said she now wished she'd started using it sooner, but she also accepted that she wasn't in that place in herself to do that at the time – still fighting, struggling on, but actually being more limited as a result. After speaking to her at the meeting I really felt positive for a while. I discussed it with Diana and she was encouraged by what I was saying, and how I was saying it. But she does think I should seriously think about using a chair.'

'Mhmm, so it left you feeling quite positive about the idea?'

'Yes, so we are both going to look at what she has – well, Diana has to come to take me there – but she was very positive about it. It's a lot to think about and, well, it may be different for me. But it was the way she described the places they could go to. How much more she could get around. She said how previously she might have struggled her way round – bit like me – but more often than not she stayed in the car.'

'Is that how it is for you, then?'

'Pretty much. I don't think I'm as bad now as she was then, I mean, on good days I can walk around if I take it carefully, though I have to stay on the ground floor, and you know going round a stately home, or a museum or a gallery, or something like that, they always seem to have chairs to sit on without arms, and that's a real pain. Nothing to push myself up with. You'd think they'd realise something so obvious. People who need to sit are likely to need arms to get up.'

'Mhmm, seems obvious to me too, hadn't had cause to think about it.'

'No, you wouldn't, but I do. Anyway, I can see her point, that the wheelchair gets her into places, gets her out, and she says she feels better for it. She said how she had been getting down, spending so much time indoors. I realise that I do that, as well, and it isn't good. It does affect me.'

'Affect you?' Jim invited Pauline to say a little more with his questioning tone.

'I guess over the months, well last couple of years really, I've kind of lost some of my confidence. I feel overwhelmed outside – all the noise, the bustle, and just big spaces. I don't like big supermarkets, not that I often go in them, Diana does the shopping, but sometimes I go in and maybe have a look around before heading for the coffee shop. It's made me think that perhaps I need the chair to get me into places like that a bit more, you know, and garden centres and just, and just get out there. I think I've kind of faded a bit.'

Jim was struck by Pauline's use of the word 'faded' and he wasn't sure what she was meaning. 'Faded? Not sure what you mean by that.'

Jim invites Pauline to explain what she means, offering opportunity for her to clarify her experience and also communicating to her his interest in what she is saying, that it is important for him to understand. It says that her world is important to him.

Pauline hadn't really thought about it herself; it was a word that had just come to mind as she was speaking. She thought about what she had said. Faded. Fading away. Fading into oblivion. Fading into the background. Yes, that's it. 'Well, it's like the sense of fading into the background, becoming less visible, sort of hiding away I suppose, keeping out of sight.'

'Fading into the background, less visible, hiding away.' Jim sought to use Pauline's words and offer back what he heard her saying, allowing her freedom to choose her own direction in developing the theme.

'The hiding away part kind of stands out a bit.' She bit her lip; she felt a surge of emotion. Her eyes were welling up with tears and her throat had suddenly gone dry and a lump had appeared in it. She swallowed. 'Oh dear, that's got to me.'

'Something about hiding away has really touched something.'

She nodded, having closed her eyes, but she could feel the tears trickling out. She bit her lip again and swallowed. 'Oh dear.' She could feel the emotional build-up inside herself; it had come from nowhere but now it was very present. She began to sob, uncontrollably. She couldn't stop herself. 'Oh God . . .' She took a deep breath trying to stem the flow but it was no good.

'So many feelings about hiding away.'

Pauline nodded; she had reached for a tissue but it was soon wet. She hadn't felt quite like this, she was going to say to herself before, but she knew she probably had. But this was so overwhelming. She just felt suddenly full of emotion and so, so tearful. She had bowed her head, and had screwed up her eyes; the tears continued to flow. 'Oh dear,' she said again, and swallowed; her throat was very dry. She reached over for her glass of water and took a sip, put it back and then continued feeling the waves of emotion. She couldn't really identify them; she just was aware of suddenly feeling very fragile and very tearful.

Jim sat with her as the feelings were released. Clearly, something about hiding away had touched into an area of herself that was full of emotional sensitivity and upset. He obviously didn't know what it was and he noted a temptation to speculate but pushed that aside, keeping his focus on Pauline. He felt a wave of tenderness towards her and he expressed this by touching her arm as he had done the previous week. This time her reaction was different. She lifted her other hand across on to the back of his hand and pressed on him. 'Oh dear,' she said again, her breathing having become quite jolted, and another wave of emotion hit her and more tears.

Pauline had felt Jim's hand and she needed to hold it. It wasn't enough to feel that reassuring touch; she needed to hold on to him, to someone, something. She didn't feel solid at all. Everything felt fluid, in motion. It was like her whole body felt tearful, her whole body . . . What a weird feeling. But she couldn't think about it; the feelings were too much for thinking to take hold. Another wave of emotion, more tears, more sobs, her throat felt like she'd swallowed a hot rubber ball. She swallowed again. Again, 'Oh dear', and then, in a very broken voice broken up with short breaths, 'I keep saying that, don't I?'

'Yes, you do, and it's OK to keep saying it as long as you need to.'

Her voice was still broken up with short intakes of breath. 'There doesn't seem much else to say at the moment.'

'Mhmm. It's OK.'

Sometimes a comment like 'it's OK' can be helpful, but it is always a danger that in fact it is completely missing the client's reality which, as in this case, is very much one of not being OK.

He gave her arm a reassuring but gentle squeeze. Immediately the flow of tears increased and Pauline's pressure on his own hand increased. She tried to take a deep breath but it became very difficult and she let the air back out, returning to shallower breaths. She couldn't get that damned rubber ball out of her throat. More emotions, another surge of tears, another 'Oh dear', and she tightened her grip on Jim's hand again.

Jim sat quietly. Something was being released and he desperately wanted to ensure he did not in any way hinder this or take Pauline away from it.

Again, the person-centred counsellor trusts the client's process. Or perhaps we should say that he trusts the client who is in process. His role is to be there for her, with her, a non-judgemental companion, accepting of what has become expressed, attentive and respectful to the client's needs and vulnerability at a time of emotional release.

Pauline was glad Jim was there, that she was not alone. She felt she might drown if she was on her own, drown in her own tears. Still that sensation, like her whole body was crying. She had the thought that if she could have released tears through her skin then she would. That image somehow became clear in her mind. She decided she wanted to try and describe it to Jim; she wanted him, someone, to hear what it was like, what she was experiencing. 'I feel like my whole body wants to cry, like I could cry through my skin.' Her voice was quite quiet and still quite broken with her short, shallow breaths.

'Your whole body could cry tears through your skin.'

Pauline nodded in a short, sharp manner; she was still feeling wave after wave of emotion. She felt drained by it, absolutely drained by it. She reached for another sip of water, rather unsteadily, took a few sips. It was cool and she needed to feel that in her throat. She took a rather unsteady deep breath and blew the air out. She felt like the emotions were subsiding a little. She took another sip and returned the glass to the table. She closed her eyes and blinked, dabbing them once more with a tissue. She blew out another deep breath. 'What was that about?'

'I was so struck by what you just said about your whole body wanting to cry.'

Pauline nodded, but that really was how it felt. 'Like my skin was crying, my muscles were crying, my . . .' She suddenly looked wide-eyed straight at Jim. 'I was about to say "my nerves are crying".' She went silent for a moment. 'My body crying out, is that possible? Can my body cry, I mean, what does that mean? But that was what it felt like. My whole body was . . .' She stopped again to think. Her head was clearing a bit now. She shook her head slightly. 'Hiding away . . .' She took a deep breath and could feel those emotions close once again. Her eyes had watered again. She swallowed once more and took a deep breath. 'I think I've just had, what do you call it, catharsis or something?'

Jim nodded. 'I think you have as well. How are you feeling?'

'Wobbly, fragile, not so tearful, but I do feel washed out by it.' She moved a little in her chair; she had been sitting slightly forward for some while and she was aware of how stiff and painful her back was, and just above her hips. She stretched and she felt a crack in her neck. It felt good to move.

'OK, so take your time to kind of be with yourself.'

Pauline nodded. 'Yes, I do need time, that was intense. That really was intense. Phew! And I feel a little calmer now, in fact, I feel very calm, and still. I mean, the feelings were overwhelming but they weren't – how can I put it – sort of heavy. No, that's not the word. I don't know how to describe them.'

'Heavy's not the word, but it's hard to really get hold of those feelings in words.'

'It is. The waves were gentle but persistent, like a large swell rather than huge waves crashing down.'

Jim had an image now. 'So, like being in the water and the swell rises up and drops, gentle but unstoppable.' The 'gentle but unstoppable' were very much his own words; they came to him as he recalled what it was like being in the sea and feeling the swell rising up and threatening to overwhelm you as it took your feet off the bottom.

'It was like a swell that started, well, it got to the point of feeling like it was passing up and through my whole body, that's why I said about feeling like my whole body wanted to cry. The feeling was everywhere.'

'The emotion rising up and down throughout your body.'

'It's still not far away. It's like I know it's there, but it isn't overwhelming me. Like I know it could rise up again. Do you think it will?'

Jim felt it appropriate to respond directly but allow Pauline as well an opportunity to explore it. 'It could, I guess, and that must leave you with thoughts and feelings about it.'

'It does. I was glad you were here, Jim. The thought of it happening if I was on my own . . .' Pauline didn't relish that prospect one little bit.

'Maybe it happened because I was here. I think sometimes our – what do we call it – our own being has a kind of wisdom. Maybe in some way it took advantage of the opportunity. I don't know, that may sound weird.' Jim was very aware he had just slid into speculation on the process and wasn't anywhere near Pauline's frame of reference.

Sometimes it is therapeutically helpful to reflect on the process with a client. It can help to develop a mutual understanding of what has been going on. However, it is important that this should not cut across the actual experience itself as it is occurring. And the interest in doing this should be raised by the client, not the counsellor taking it into their head to tell the client what they think has taken place.

'Maybe. Maybe.' Pauline was back with that sensation of her whole body wanting to cry. That feeling was persisting. It wasn't that she felt like her whole body did want to cry, not at this moment, but she could still feel the sensation that was present when it had happened during that episode a few minutes earlier.

'I'm still with that sense of how I felt when my whole body wanted to cry. In fact, in a way I think it was, it did, the emotion was everywhere, the sensations . . . I've never felt anything quite like that.' Pauline was shaking her head and looking at Jim.

'Do you want to explore that – it sounds like you do – what was that sensation of your whole body crying all about?' Jim realised that maybe he could have worded that better and just added something along the lines of the sense 'of your whole body crying'.

'It was like I was in mourning.' Pauline paused. 'I'm not sure why I said that, but yes, like my body was in mourning.'

'In mourning. Your whole body was in mourning.'

Pauline nodded. 'I think my body was in mourning for itself, and I know that must sound weird, but that's what it seemed like. My whole body, mourning its loss, grieving.' Pauline could still feel that calmness still very present. And though she felt tired, it was a different sort of tired. There was energy as well, a kind of gentle energy. It actually felt good.

'Yes, I can appreciate what you are saying, that the mourning wasn't just in your head, or your heart, your whole body was experiencing it and you were experiencing it throughout your body.'

'That's a nice way of putting it. Yes, like my body feels something and I then feel my body feeling it. I like that. Fits with how I see things. I don't think of myself as just my body, it's not what I believe. I do see myself, and I hope this doesn't sound too weird, but like we have fields of energy and I have an emotional field and a mental field and somewhere deeper a kind of spiritual field. And, you know, what I felt just now seemed to be like I really felt my emotional field and yet it also felt very tangible and in my body as well.'

'Like you have a field of emotion and you experienced its presence in your body?'

'Yes, it was weird, I mean it was kind of physical but it wasn't. It's so hard to describe. But it really did feel like my whole body crying, in mourning for a loss, its loss.'

'The act of mourning became present for you across your whole body. That's how I'm hearing what you are saying. Is that right?'

'Yes. It wasn't like me mourning my loss, it really felt like my body mourning its loss.' Pauline could feel herself in awe of what had happened and how she was making sense of it. 'Could that be?'

'It's what you experienced?' Jim wanted to help Pauline stay with her own evaluation of what had occurred.

'Yes and, you know, something has shifted for me, there's no doubt about that.' She was aware of tiredness coming back at her again. It was odd. She still felt the vitality that seemed to have emerged after the release, but she could also feel tiredness, particularly in her eyes. She yawned and glanced at the clock. Just a few minutes left.

The session drew to a close. Jim checked out how Pauline was feeling; he was caught between feeling concerned as to whether she might be overwhelmed again, and wanting to trust that she would be able to cope with it. He knew it was his anxiety, but he did just check that Diana was going to be around for a while. Pauline confirmed that she was.

If Pauline was still distressed, still in the midst of an emotional release and finding herself unable to contain or control it, what would the counsellor then do, particularly when counselling someone in their home with the possibility that there may not be anyone around after they left? Perhaps asking if there was a friend that could come round, or a close relative, might be appropriate in such circumstances.

After Jim left, Pauline sat for a few moments thinking, before Diana came in. 'You OK?'

Pauline nodded. 'Yes. I've just had the most amazing experience.'

'Oh yes?' Diana raised a quizzical eyebrow.

'No, I mean a really amazing experience.' She went on to describe what had happened. It felt good talking about it and as she spoke her tiredness began to lift again. She knew she felt different. She couldn't really describe it, not clearly, but she sensed it. She knew that when she visited Isabel she had been in a very different place in herself, maybe more receptive to what she would have to say and show her. She didn't know. But she was excited about seeing what she had, and that was quite a new experience – being excited at the thought of looking at someone else's wheelchairs!

Jim sat outside in his car; he was wiped out and he was buzzing. That was intense, he thought to himself, and he was glad he had another supervision session the next day. I need to unload some of this, he thought to himself, talk it through, clarify myself on the process and my process. He knew he had to be affected by their encounter and while at this moment he wasn't at all sure how he had been affected, he felt that he could check himself out in supervision. He was self-aware enough to know that just because you didn't have a direct sense of how you had been affected by a client didn't mean that you hadn't been affected. He saw so many professionals in other areas of healthcare who were blind to the emotional impact that their work had on them, and it affected the way they were with their patients or clients, with family and friends. He was grateful that he was working in a profession that saw supervision as a fundamental, professional requirement. It helped keep him psychologically, emotionally and mentally healthy – all of which contributed to his physical well-being – and helped to ensure he could be more fully present and therapeutically helpful with his clients.

Points for discussion

- Evaluate the accuracy of Jim's empathy and its therapeutic impact during these sessions.
- How would you account for the emergence of the 'anxious me' and 'accepting me' parts of Pauline in terms of person-centred theory?
- What impact did the two sessions have on you? What thoughts and feelings became present for you and how might they impact on working with Pauline if you were her counsellor?
- How do you prepare yourself for seeing clients?
- What role did Jim's unconditional positive regard have in enabling Pauline to connect with her sense of mourning?
- What would you do if your client was deeply emotionally distressed at the end of a session and you were concerned about leaving them on their own at home?
- Write your own notes for these sessions.

CHAPTER 7

Supervision session 2: respect for the client

'I need to spend some time processing my experience with Pauline yesterday, the client who is struggling with whether or not she should use a wheelchair?'

David nodded. 'The way you said that seems to communicate that it was quite powerful. You sounded quite overwhelmed somehow.' David had noted that there was a certain quietness to Jim's voice, as if he had just come through something extremely draining.

'It was overwhelming. Pauline had a major, I guess you'd call it cathartic, episode. She really connected with something deep, some very body-centred feelings.'

'Body-centred?'

'She talked about her whole body wanting to cry; she used some incredibly powerful images, of her skin wanting to ... I can't recall exactly how she said it, but like it wanted to cry, like tears coming through her skin. And she talked of feeling as if she, her body, was in mourning, mourning for the losses, you know, loss of mobility, loss of pain-free existence, I guess, though I don't recall we ever got to anything specific like that. It was more general.'

'So her whole body wanting to cry?'

'And so much emotion, so much seemed to be present for her. She described it as if she had a field of emotion and it was all feeling so much.' Jim could recall vividly now how it had been, sitting with her, holding her arm. He remembered her saying 'Oh dear' again and again as the waves of feeling surged through her.

'So much emotion, and how was it for you listening to her, attending to her?'

'I felt quite calm and at the same time was feeling the enormity of what was happening for Pauline. The way she described it, I hadn't heard someone talk quite that way before. Her whole body in mourning image was so, well, tangible, you know? And, well, it really made sense given that she has got MS problems in much of her body. There was something that just felt right about her whole body feeling like that.'

David nodded. 'I'm also aware of feeling the enormity of it and I am hearing about it second hand, as it were. I am aware of what I am feeling listening to you, and that is something about feeling my focus is sharpened up and it makes me feel alert. I am wondering whether that has any relevance to your experience.'

David uses his own experience of his reactions to what Jim is saying to try and inform what else may be present for Jim. This can be a valuable approach in supervision. The supervisor can connect with feelings and thoughts that, while not consciously present for the counsellor, do represent something significant for the therapeutic relationship they have with their client.

Jim thought about it. 'Yes, I was very much alert, and thinking about it, I was sitting on the padded stool in that session – I'd moved closer to her in the previous session when she was distressed, and used the stool all through that last session. Thinking back to it, my body was quite rigid, and I was quite stiff afterwards.' Jim thought about it a bit more. Yes, he really had been focused during that emotional release, and he remembered what Pauline had said about fields of emotion. He found himself wondering how that might have affected him. 'I've just remembered something else. Pauline talked of her belief that she had an emotional field, that they weren't simply by-products of chemical reactions. I'm just wondering how, if that's the case, her field of emotion might impact on my own.'

'Mhmm. So, the focus left you feeling stiff but that could have been the seating position. You felt focused, alert, and then this notion of a field of emotion impacting on you.' David was aware of this idea, but he left it open for Jim to follow up with what was present for him.

'Quite tense as well.' Jim thought for a moment. He wanted to say something more. 'I do think feeling gets across; I'm sure I pick up on my client's experience in some way, tune in, particularly in those really deep moments, but maybe it is happening all the time?'

'Maybe. If true – and I agree that this may be happening, we have to be at least open to the possibility – then it really does have implications for the nature, purpose, role, impact of therapeutic relationship – both on the client and the counsellor.'

'Makes me think of just how important those core conditions are, and how we need to be authentic.' Jim was reflecting back to the experience with Pauline. He was back with that sense of calmness that had been present for him as well. 'I'm also aware of that calmness, and can feel it being very present as we are discussing this now.'

'Interesting, that you felt tense and you were also saying you felt calm, and that calmness is present.'

Jim was nodding thoughtfully. Yes, he had felt calm, he was feeling calm, and yet … Where was the tension he had felt? He tried to think back to the session. He could suddenly see Pauline very clearly again talking about feeling her nerves wanted to cry, yes, that was it, her nerves, her body, her muscles, her skin wanted to cry. He noted he was taking a deep breath and felt a wave of sadness within himself. It was quite intense and took him by surprise.

David noted the look of surprise on Jim's face and commented, 'Feelings?'

'I just suddenly went back to something Pauline had said, she'd begun saying, before talking about her whole body being in mourning, about her nerves wanting to cry, her muscles wanting to cry, like it was her diseased body wanting to release so much. And I'm aware I'm in touch with some really strong feelings of sadness just at the moment.' Jim went back into silence as he felt more the presence of the sadness within him. It felt ... He wasn't sure, but it wasn't a surging sadness, more gentle, calm, but very present, very present. Hard to locate exactly. He was aware his own eyes were watering. 'That sadness is really present for me, David, really present. I need to be with this and see where it leads. But it feels almost as though I'm experiencing some kind of, I don't know, sympathetic reaction to what Pauline experienced. I mean sympathetic in the sense that it feels like ...' He paused again; he knew he wasn't sure how to describe what he was feeling. 'Guess I really made a connection. It's like it just makes so much sense for a person to feel the way Pauline was feeling. But I wonder how many people are that sensitive.'
'Seems that maybe you are, Jim, it really has touched you.'

Rather than empathise with Jim's comment, David brings the focus into Jim's own experience and reaction, into the here and now. By holding Jim in this way, and in effect not allowing him to speculate on the sensitivity of others, he offers opportunity to further explore his reaction. However, Jim isn't there. He's still with his own thoughts and wondering about how others might be carrying similar feelings locked up inside of themselves, locked in their bodies.

Jim continued to sit with the feeling of sadness that had become very present for him. And he was aware that his thoughts were not just focused on Pauline; rather, he was thinking about just how many people must have this kind of reality yet which hasn't broken into their awareness, how many people are in a sense walking around in bodies that are crying out, but aren't heard. Yet, at the same time, Jim was thinking that it was such a weird way of thinking about things, and part of him felt that it was too way-out. And yet ... Another deep breath and he began to speak, but not before he had shaken his head a few times. 'I guess that in a way I've been put in touch with my own bodily awareness to some degree, and yet I have nothing to compare to Pauline. But it does leave me wondering, you know, just what may be present within our bodily experience which somehow does not reach consciousness. And what that's all about.' Jim noted that the sadness was lifting, that he was beginning to feel ... the only word that made any sense was 'liberated' from what he had been experiencing. Then he realised that, of course, for someone like Pauline there was unlikely to be any liberation, not in life anyway. He pursed his lips. 'I'm beginning to wonder how this may all be affecting my empathy, David.'
'That these feelings could be affecting how you empathise?'

'I didn't feel blocked in the session and so maybe it is just where I am in myself now, but I realise that we never really got into what her body was really mourning for. There was just this cathartic release.'

'You sound like you feel that there should have been more insight?'

Hearing David put it like that, Jim knew instinctively that his response was 'no'. 'It's not like that. No, I mean, I guess I'd have been interested to know, yes, that's it, I'm sure it's my own curiosity, but it wasn't something Pauline got into, and we were heading towards the end of the session anyway. But that's my need to know. Maybe at some level Pauline does know, perhaps she is very aware and chose not to go down that route.' Jim felt sure that it was his curiosity and he was mindful that while that was a good quality for a counsellor, it could become extreme and be simply just plain nosy. He didn't feel it was that; more he felt he needed to connect with what was happening for Pauline. It intrigued him. He glanced at the clock and was aware that the supervision session was passing. And he had other matters he wanted to raise.

> It is fascinating how much can arise from counselling. So much time could be spent in supervision processing it, and yet there is a time constraint to this. While one has to be practical, the truth is that generally speaking one could always use more supervision time to explore the counselling process, the impact on the counsellor, the effect of the counsellor's responses on the client and the experience of bringing the session's therapeutic content into the supervisory relationship.

'I'm feeling clearer, it's been good to air this and speculate a bit, and I can recognise and own my curiosity, and that may help me allow Pauline to choose her own focus next session.'

'That's important, don't forget, she will have a week to live with that experience as well, and it will have been more real, more pertinent for her than for you, and she will make of it what she will. She needs to be allowed the freedom to make her own sense of it and to integrate the experience and the meaning she attaches to it. It sounds incredibly profound and I am sure it has had, and is having, a significant impact on her. But what that will be, who knows?'

'I know that I don't know. But I'm so glad it happened.' Jim paused. 'I also wanted to just highlight another thing that emerged during the sessions, I think it was the previous one. There was something about Pauline experiencing anxiety about the possibility of having to accept using a wheelchair, and what it would mean. She really does fear losing her own mobility so much, and I can appreciate that. And she also spoke of an acceptance as well?'

'Acceptance? Of being in a wheelchair?'

'Sort of. She said something about it being quite a calm place inside herself, a sort of place where it was OK, but that her sense was that her anxiety kept her away from that place, that it was somehow dangerous? She didn't say that, it's my own impression as I sit here now and talk about it.'

'Like it's dangerous to accept it?'

'Like it's OK to accept it but there is a danger in allowing that acceptance to dominate. It's like her anxious self wants to keep her independent and on her own two feet at virtually any cost.'

'Which is very often the response in these situations.'

'And she recognises this. She sees it as a battle and each time she has to give something up it is like a retreat, ready to kind of group to fight to cope at the next level of disability. But I guess I was struck by this struggle between the two and how she could sense this calm acceptance but ... oh yes, I think she said something about when she finds that place then it triggers the anxiety again.'

'Like the anxiety becomes a reaction to or against acceptance?'

'That's right. In a way it was confusing and I guess I wanted to talk it out, try to order it in my own head because I'm sure we will come back to this. The notion that the structure of self is composed of 'configurations' [Mearns, 1999], well, I'm sure it has application.' Another thought was with Jim. 'And as I say this I am struck by the sense that at some level, or in some part of herself, Pauline knows that it will be OK to use a wheelchair. But to this other part of her structure of self that is so dangerous.'

'So there is something about this other part, possibly her anxious part but not necessarily, there could be another part, but there is something about this other part that presumably feels very threatened, very threatened, and gives Pauline an experience to take her away from it.'

'From what is threatening her?'

'Maybe, but it could be something that is simply threatening to that part of her self.'

'Like the part of her that, for instance, might want to preserve independence or feel in control.'

'Could be. Could be all kinds of things and obviously while we can speculate we cannot bring this into the session and start trying to hypothesise as to what parts exist.'

'I know. These parts are very much the client's experience and it is for Pauline to identify what they are through her own, I guess, self-experience.' Jim thought for a moment. 'The prospect of being in a wheelchair must challenge so many beliefs, notions, concepts that a person has about themselves. I'm struck as I sit here by the enormity of it. I mean, I kind of knew it at a sort of intellectual level and had a sense of the emotional impact it has on people, but it absolutely, well, it's like almost throwing a hand grenade into someone's structure of self. It's mind blowing.'

David was nodding. He hadn't quite thought of it this way, and found himself responding, 'Literally – and emotions too.'

They both lapsed into silence – each, in their own way, having connected with something that was suddenly very real, very present and very awesome.

In supervision it can be important to in a very real sense honour the client for what they are going through. Sometimes the recounting of sessions, the therapeutic speculation, the exploration of the quality and nature of the therapeutic relationship is called to a halt by a moment of respectful silence for a client. Holding this kind of respectful silence, acknowledging the immensity of what a client is passing through, is important. In our busy, busy world we can lose sight of the need for this time, rushing on to talk about the next client. Counsellors, and supervisors, need to share silences when they arise in the context of their exploration of the work being done with a client – taking time to be with what, as in this case, has become suddenly very real, very present and very awesome.

It was Jim who broke the silence. 'And it makes me think of how many people come through this experience, adapt, adjust and emotionally and mentally survive, and in fact grow through this experience. And I guess many do not as well.'

David was thinking of the Chinese glyph for, what was it, crisis. He'd read about it years ago, that it was composed of two other glyphs, one for danger, the other for opportunity. Seemed to sum it up. He shared his remembering with Jim.

Jim responded. 'Yes, I'd come across that. And it does have a lot of meaning for these kinds of situation. But it isn't just mobility that is in danger in Pauline's mind; it is the different parts of her sense of self, or that make up her sense of self, which are being threatened or challenged. I'm kind of tempted to say that she knows it won't stop her mobility, but it will affect her independence if her leg muscles weaken, or even her joints may stiffen from reduced usage, and that's a big fear for her.'

'Yes, and there is also the fact of how she will feel being viewed as a person in a wheelchair rather than standing upright.'

'Fear of the "does she take sugar" syndrome?'

'Partly that, but what it means to her as, well, as a woman. There are going to be so many aspects of all of this that she may want or need to work on. It could be really long-term work, you know, if that is what Pauline wants.'

'Time will tell on that. My sense is that she may – but then she may, if she gets to the point of deciding to accept the wheelchair, decide that that's enough. She's come to terms with it enough to get on with her life.'

'And we must trust her in that; she will know her needs and what is uppermost for her.'

Jim thought for a moment. 'We can "over-therapise", can't we? We can get so caught up in all the emotional implications, and helping a client untangle or get clarity about their structure of self, that we can forget that perhaps the client simply wants to have space to come to a decision and, having made their decision, move on and make the best of it, whatever it might be.'

'We have to be ready to accept that, but also aware that for some people they will want to work more deeply and extensively, and so we offer them that. But as a person-centred therapist you/we are not going to push them either way, of course.'

'No, but you can appreciate the temptation to cling to clients and in effect push them on a psychological journey that is the desire of the therapist more than that of the client.'

'And that has to be watched for and, well, hopefully supervision will pick that up.'

'You know, I think more and more people are wary of that. I think there is a more goal-oriented sense among people these days. They have a problem, they want it sorted.'

'But often they want relief of symptoms, and they can get that with a short period of counselling maybe, or prescribed medication . . .'

'Or something more illicit, or, of course, alcohol.'

'. . . but it takes time to really adjust to these kind of life changes, like Pauline is facing, and to do so in a way that is healthy for her structure of self. It puts it under a lot of strain, and yet, as we know, it can be the making, or prove the breaking, of people.'

'Yeah.' He thought of Pauline. Her sense was that she was a fighter, that whatever happened, she would continue being herself, even if she had to go around on wheels. In a funny kind of way, he suddenly got the sense that it might make her even more formidable – no longer so drained by the constant physical, emotional and mental struggle to keep mobile, and able to move around more easily. But she had a huge adjustment to make. He wanted to help her in that, if that was her choice. He kind of felt it would be, but he knew that it was up to her. There was an inevitability about it, simply more a matter of time, of when rather than if. When the time is right for her, when she is ready to embrace change – or was it truer to say when change embraced her?

The moment when such change arrives will be a 'turning point'. Such a moment has been described in the *I Ching*: 'There is movement but it is not brought about by force . . . The movement is natural, arising spontaneously. For this reason the transformation of the old becomes easy. The old is discarded and the new is introduced. Both measures accord with the time; therefore no harm results.' (Wilhelm, 1968, p. 97)

Jim was left feeling a huge sense of respect for Pauline. And as he connected with that feeling he remembered that moment the session before last where their eyes had met, that moment of real, deep, calm connection. He described it to David.

'Made a deep impression, you felt calm, you say?'

'Very calm, very steady, a real moment of meeting, you know?'

'And I just wonder how important that moment was for what followed in the next session. Maybe there was something communicated in that moment that allowed her feelings – the emotions, that sense of her body wanting to cry – to happen in your presence.' David smiled. 'I'm really touched by the work you are doing, Jim, and I have a real sense of how connected you are. I guess, and I'm putting a supervisor hat on here, I guess I need to say keep space for yourself. And I am aware that it is a need to say it, a professional need, while at the same time I feel and know that you will.'

Jim smiled. 'I'm glad you put it like that. Yes, I appreciate your supervisory concern and your personal belief in what I am doing.' He was nodding his head. 'Yes, that feels good, and, yes, I am aware that this is powerful stuff and, well, you'll be hearing more about it, that's for sure.'

'Yes. Didn't Rogers write of people as process persons, or something like that?'

'I'm not sure, but it sounds like something he might have said, or written.'

'Well, Pauline's in process – and so are you – and they are running parallel and have a point of contact once a week in which you, while mindful of your process, maintain an attending focus on her process. Trust it, I'm sure you will. She may take a long time on her decision, it may happen fast. But we have to be sure that it is hers and that she is clear in herself about it.'

David knew he was speaking from his own sense of how people could make decisions which were not thought through, or out of the reaction to a part of themselves that was not the whole person and left them feeling – eventually – dissatisfied with the decision they had taken. The more self-aware Pauline became, the greater the likelihood that decisions she made would be right for her, even though there were always likely to be parts of herself that would have some doubts. But sometimes, so long as you knew what they were and were clear about their origin, they could be accepted as relevant but not be allowed to dominate the choice.

The session moved on to another client of Jim's. He was grateful for the discussion they had had. It had opened up his thinking and his feeling about Pauline, himself and what was happening in the therapeutic process. He often wondered at how much material could emerge from a couple of counselling sessions. The complexity of people and of relationships never ceased to amaze him. And yet, he thought to himself, we find our way through it. Yes, making mistakes, but hopefully learning from them. So much complexity, and yet . . . He felt himself smiling as he drove home later, reflecting on the supervision session, and yet it is all so simple. If only we could truly understand the meaning of love – non-possessive, unconditional love.

He hit the brake; he'd been so much in his thoughts he hadn't noticed the red traffic light. Bloody hell, he thought to himself, his heart was racing – love is all very well, but you still have to keep your wits about you!

Counselling session 5: positive feelings, anxious reactions

Pauline had had quite a week. She had been to see the person who had the motorised vehicle – it seemed more like that than a wheelchair – and she had

had a go with it, and found it quite good to drive, though she wasn't sure if it gave her back enough support. However, she was pleased and had come back quite enthusiastic about it. She was telling Jim about it. 'You know, it was really smooth and it felt kind of substantial. I mean, I've experienced ordinary wheelchairs and, well, they feel very much like what they are, but this felt somehow so much more solid. I felt more secure thinking back to it, you know.'

'Mhmm, something secure for you about the solidity of it.'

'Yes, and I realise now how important that is. Something about feeling vulnerable in an ordinary chair. Most of the powered ones I've seen have small wheels, and maybe they're not all like that, but it seemed limiting somehow and I could see myself getting stuck. So I left feeling quite positive, in fact, I could see myself using it and, well, it did seem like a good idea. But . . .'

As she said that last word Jim noticed that the expression on her face had changed. From looking quite positive and upbeat now Pauline suddenly appeared uncertain once more. Jim reflected back her comment and empathised with what he sensed was present through her facial expression. 'But . . . and you look so uncertain.'

'I am. I got the panics last night and I don't think I've really got over them. I mean I just sort of lost it, you know, I mean really lost it. I had been feeling so positive with the idea, and really felt like I had made a decision. And then, wham! From nowhere – well, actually from inside me. I just started feeling really, really anxious and all these thoughts kept running through my head.' She paused.

'Mhmm, so many thoughts . . .'

'And I just got myself really worked up. I mean, it's not the money, I can afford it, you know, and it would be so useful to buzz around in locally. And yes, we could get a converted car to take it as well, though I'd be better off with a powered wheelchair for that, and somehow it was the "what do I get?", "what do I do?", and it just spun out of control. And I'm still very close to it all even now.'

'So you got really panicky, it's close now, and I'm hearing that it was around choice – just what do you get?'

Pauline nodded. 'I really liked what Isabel had and, yes, it would be handy, but I can also see that a powered wheelchair could be more useful. I mean, the other was too big for indoors, and for a converted car, and then, well, I kind of guess I began to see how maybe a powered wheelchair would be more practical, and probably more supportive for my back as well, and then I just got all panicky and anxious. I was in tears yesterday evening. I felt . . . I don't know, I kind of felt trapped.'

'Trapped?'

'Trapped by, well, thinking I knew what I wanted and then realising maybe it wasn't. And then I was back to thinking about an ordinary powered wheelchair and then I lost it. I couldn't see how to make a decision, and I began to think that what I had sort of thought would be so great actually wouldn't be so practical for me.' Pauline could feel the emotions close once again, but she swallowed them back down. She was feeling determined that she wanted to discuss her options rather than experience another bout of emoting; she'd been doing that and it hadn't resolved anything.

'So feeling stuck, unable to make a decision, but realising that the larger motorised buggy would be too cumbersome?' Jim wasn't sure if his empathic understanding was quite accurate, hence the questioning tone.

'I'd really felt I wanted it, I could see myself using it, but now, I don't know. I mean, oh God, I just get so panicky and anxious and then I can't think straight and . . . I don't know what to do.' She was looking down and her voice had lowered towards the end of her sentence.

'Seems like you'd really lifted your hopes, really made a decision, and then suddenly it's like, you're questioning it, and so anxious that it's hard to think straight.'

Pauline continued to sit looking down. She was feeling drained by it all. She had realised, talking to Isabel, how much she used both her forms of transport, but she knew she had only really wanted to think about the outdoor one. It didn't look like a wheelchair. She didn't want to look like she was in a wheelchair. She knew that; it had come clear to her more and more. She wanted to be upright, however wobbly and painful it was, however much it took out of her. And yet she didn't want that as well. She liked the idea of sitting down and moving around. Isabel had offered her the opportunity to sit in the powered wheelchair but she had declined. She should have realised then that she was putting all her emphasis on the other motorised scooter – at least, that's what it seemed like to her, just had extra wheels. She could ride a scooter, she could think of herself riding a kind of scooter. That wasn't the same as a wheelchair. She had so many thoughts in her head as she sat there, not knowing what to do, how to resolve it. And being so aware that her emotions were threatening to break out any moment, and she so wanted to keep them at bay, to try and keep a rational focus. But it was difficult . . . so difficult. She could feel her stomach tighten and her throat begin to get dry and hot, and her eyes were beginning to water. She closed them and felt tears trickling down her cheeks. She swallowed, opened her eyes, reached over to her glass of water and took a sip. No, she wasn't going to let her feelings wash over her today. She dried her eyes and her cheeks.

'I just blanked the wheelchair, it must have been so obvious. Actually, Diana told me that was what I had done, but I got angry and denied it. She was right, of course. But we had a row about it. But I admitted to it last night. I was only fooling myself. It's not just about the fear of losing the strength in my legs, but that is important. It's also about being seen in a wheelchair, you know, that's big, that's so big.' Pauline lapsed back into silence.

Jim was nodding and thinking back to that last supervision session. So much adjustment within Pauline to come to terms with what may be inevitable. He put his thoughts aside and responded to what he understood her to be saying. 'Fooling yourself, yeah, and you don't want to lose the strength in your legs, but you sure don't want to be seen in a wheelchair.' As Jim said it he wondered just how much of Pauline felt that way, and he guessed quite a large and dominant part, at least at this moment.

Pauline listened to Jim, to what he had said. *Fooling herself*, yeah, her words, but hearing them being said back – who was she fooling? She was going to need a wheelchair that gave her support and she knew it and she fucking hated it and she could do fuck all about it. Left her feeling angry with herself.

> The anger at herself has emerged. She knows she is avoiding the wheelchair, not wanting to accept that reality. She hates knowing she's fooling herself, but she now realises that is exactly what she has been doing. It's suddenly much more clear to her, and she hates it, and she probably doesn't really want to own it, she's still fighting it, but maybe has realised she is losing the battle as she sees it.

'I'm only fooling myself, Jim, I'm only fooling myself.' She spoke slowly and with a tone of resignation, almost sarcasm.

'Only yourself.'

'Fuck it, why can't I bloody well accept it, but I can't, I have to fight it, I have to.' Her voice had increased in volume and she had closed her eyes again. She continued, but she spoke more quietly now. 'But I can't fight it, not really. It's just that I'm only 53, if I go into a wheelchair now, I mean, it could be years, years . . .' Her voice tailed off. Pauline could just see years stretching ahead of her, losing her strength, becoming more and more reliant on Diana, until, who knows, she wouldn't be able to cope any more. And then what? Then what? It felt pretty damned bleak. She could feel herself knotting up again at the thought of it. She heard Jim 'mhmming' in response to what she had said. There wasn't much else to say, really. That was how it was. She knew she had to come to terms with it, but that didn't stop her hating it, and fearing it.

'Can't accept it, have to fight it, but you can't really fight it, some part of you knows that.'

'I think more and more of me knows that. There's a fighter in me, and sometimes I think I'm still fighting but the battle's already lost. But I keep fighting, you know – remember that Japanese guy who they found decades after the war had finished, still thinking it was going on?' She had stopped speaking and was shaking her head. 'That's me, somehow, still fighting. No one told me to stop fighting. No one told me to start getting used to something different. That's what I have to do now. That's the battle ahead of me, adjusting, adapting.' Pauline paused again; that air of resignation, of defeat, had entered into her voice.

'Adjusting, adapting.' Words of a song came to Jim's mind, he couldn't recall where from – 'the battle's lost, the war is won'. 'Words of a song have come to mind and, well, feels relevant somehow. Makes me think that maybe a battle's been lost but there's still a war to be won.'

'That's easy to say.' Pauline could feel herself flaring up at Jim. 'Easy for you to say, anyway.' There was a real edge to her voice. Jim could feel the change of atmosphere.

'Yeah, too easy.' He didn't try to defend what he had said; what was the point? It had been in his frame of reference and wasn't something that Pauline wanted to hear, or felt able to hear.

So much anger has risen to the surface for Pauline. Her feeling good about the motorised buggy or scooter was a hope to avoid the wheelchair. But she is moving inexorably towards the realisation of the inevitability of it. And she's angry with herself, with the world, and now with Jim for the stupid thing he'd said.

Pauline appreciated that Jim had then responded how he had. Somehow it felt good to know he was human, got it wrong. 'I'm sorry. I'm frustrated and angry and still don't know what to do.'

'And I guess the last thing you need is me quoting words of songs at you. Can't say I blame you. And yeah, anger, frustration, feeling stuck and a stupid counsellor.'

'No. Not at all. Thanks for being human!' She paused before continuing, 'I really felt so good going over to Isabel's and everything, and afterwards, but it was last night. I guess I saw things more clearly again and I didn't like it. I hate thinking of the future, of my future.' As she finished speaking Pauline realised that her jaw had tightened. She was suddenly feeling a fresh wave of determination, not that she knew where it had come from. 'I can't keep thinking like this. It doesn't do me any good. I've got to make a decision and get on with it. I've got to do something, go for it, and make the most of it. I'm going to have to get a powered wheelchair, I know that, and I'm going to have to get used to it and learn to appreciate it, be grateful for it. It'll make things easier, but I have got to keep walking as well. I can't just spend all my time in it.'

'That all sounds very powerful and affirming, Pauline. A real determination.'

'I've always been determined, but then, when I can see a way ahead then that's how I am. I go for it. I weigh things up and when I am clear about what to do, then that's it. But I'd lost touch with it.'

Jim noted her use of the past tense. 'And now you are feeling back in touch?'

'I've got to be. The only other way is down, and I'm not going to let that happen.'

'You're not going down, you're determined not to let that happen.'

'I am. I'm not sure how I suddenly started to feel this way, and it doesn't matter. Talking to you helps.'

'It was me recalling the words from that song that fired you up, I think.' Jim felt he was taking a risk reminding Pauline of that, but it did feel like that had contributed. And the next line had just come into his mind; 'I think we've cleared the air.' Pauline was speaking again before he had a chance to decide whether to share this.

'It wasn't the words, and it wasn't my reaction. Well it was, I mean, made me realise I had to get my act together. Guess that independent bit of me, you know, sort it yourself, don't rely on someone else. So many contradictions in all of this. It's like I have to learn to use parts of me in different ways. I mean, my independent streak has been a big part of me struggling to keep walking, you know, and suddenly, here I am thinking of that part of me in relation to getting used to accepting and using a wheelchair.'

Yes, Jim thought, there'll be a lot of that. 'Seems like that is a big part of the battle, like being you but focusing your energies in a new direction.'

That made sense to Pauline. 'Yes.'

Jim didn't mention the other words from the song. They had come to mind at that previous moment, but the moment had passed. Sometimes in counselling we may feel an urge to say something that feels relevant to the therapeutic process; however, we may not get a chance to voice it. We have to let go of it. However, where something persists then it may need voicing, though in a way that conveys the counsellor's ownership of their experience, thought or feeling.

They sat in silence for a minute or two, Pauline aware of her own process of steeling herself up for what lay ahead, and mentally seeking to impose a fresh will on herself, to think the unthinkable and get on with it. She knew that the anxious part of her was around still, probably always would be for now, but she had to ignore that, she had to act. She'd been stuck trying to decide what to do for too long. She was decisive by nature and she needed to be back in touch with that side of herself. She'd lost touch with it these past few weeks. She was going to get it back.

Jim sat observing Pauline. She did seem to have more of an air of determination. He didn't know what was in her thoughts, or what she was feeling. He guessed she would share this if and when she felt like it. He stayed with her silence and waited for her to speak.

'My mind's made up. I'm going to get a powered chair for use in the home, and to get around a bit locally, and look at some kind of van I guess, or something that can take it. I've seen them advertised. I know Diana is up for it. She's always shown more enthusiasm. I think she feels trapped sometimes by how limiting it is when I'm determined to only walk anywhere when we have driven out. I've got to change that. I don't want her to push me around, though, that's not what it's about. I want my own power.'

'Mhmm, that sums something up. "I want my own power".'

'Yeah, and that's what I'm going to get. I'm going to do my research, see what's available, prices and stuff, and take action. I can afford it. I'm fortunate. I know not everyone can. I'd kind of put money away in the past for that rainy day. Well, now it's raining, you know, I need to break out. I've got myself stuck, trapped, and I needed to as well. I've needed to struggle on as I have, you know, that's me, but now I need change.'

'Yeah, you really want that change. Time to move on, to a new battle, and maybe fresh opportunity.' Jim had realised he had got that Chinese glyph in his head, the one David had mentioned in supervision – that was why he had said opportunity.

'I've got to create opportunities for myself.' Pauline moved about in her chair; she was feeling stiff, she'd been leaning slightly forward for too long. She sat back.

'Yeah, I got stuck, like my back, too fixed, and that was OK at the time, but now I must move on, accept how things are and move on.'

'I really hear the strength of that urge to move on, to break out of being stuck.' Jim kept his focus on what Pauline was saying. In the back of his mind he acknowledged a sense of how maybe parts of Pauline would still react against it, but that wasn't where she was now and his empathy was towards what she was communicating.

'Yes.' There was a power in her voice. That resignation he had heard earlier had gone. This was a different Pauline, one he hadn't really experienced before. It felt good. It felt more alive in the room, more energy. He hoped she could sustain it, and he recognised that the rollercoaster of emotion and thought could still sweep her up and down a few more times yet. 'Time for me to be a bit more positive.'

Another silence.

Pauline was aware that she did feel strong and yet she also sensed that panicky edge as well. It was curious feeling them both at the same time, but something inside her seemed to be telling her that she was stronger, that she didn't have to let the panic overtake her. She was determined not to let it happen. And yet . . . She took a deep breath and looked at Jim. 'I really have got to move on, I can't stay like this. Time is passing and I know, deep down, that I have to adapt, but I know I have to be disciplined with myself as well, keep walking on the good days and not take the chair as the easy option. I need to control it, not let it dominate me.'

'You really want to be sure that *you* are in control.'

Yes, thought Pauline, I've got to keep in control. I've got to control my feelings and reactions. She looked up towards the corner of the room, staring at it, and noted a cobweb. There was a fly caught in it, still struggling. She watched the spider moving towards it, unaffected by the web. Able to move freely. Yes, she thought, I can be like that fly, or I can be like the spider. I can either get myself stuck, or I can move freely. The wheelchair will help me move freely.

'Yeah, I guess my mind is made up. I'm sure I've still got doubts though.'

'Yes, even though you have made up your mind, there's still a part of you that's unsure.'

'But I think sometimes you have to do things in spite of yourself, I mean, regardless of reservations. It's like you have to kind of bite the bullet and go for it. And I think that's where I'm at. Go for it and make the best of it, and maybe I can find advantages from it.' Pauline stopped speaking. She was thinking about getting outside sometimes on days when it was a real struggle. But she was still sure that she would only use it on bad days. On the better days, when she could walk, then it wasn't a problem. And anyway, she did have periods of remission, although they were less frequent these days.

Jim was very aware of feeling something of the enormity of Pauline's decision. 'It feels like a huge decision, but I can also sense your focus and single-mindedness to go for it and make the best of it.'

The dialogue moved towards a consideration of the advantages of having that extra mobility on bad days. Sometimes when she was stuck indoors she really felt like she wanted to get outside, but the effort to do so just made it seem pointless; but if she was in the chair she could get out and she could get a bit of fresh air. It felt good thinking about that.

'I think I need to get it and see how it goes for a while. Use it around here and maybe outside a bit to get my confidence. It's going to be a big thing for me, though, to be seen in it. I can feel myself going just thinking about that.' Pauline was aware that this really was a big issue for her. She would have to get over it, she knew that, but it seemed like a real block.

'Mhmm, that really does affect you, the thought of being seen in a wheelchair.'

'It's like I can't imagine it, but I can. Does that make sense?'

'I think so. Like you can't kind of see yourself in a wheelchair among people, and yet in a way you kind of can? Like part of you doesn't want to imagine it?'

The last sentence wasn't necessary. The client has not introduced talking in terms of parts at this point, so why has the counsellor?

'It's hard to explain. Maybe, yes, you're right, I don't want to see myself like that. And I guess I'll continue thinking like that until I get used to it. I'm sure I will. I mean, I've got used to using sticks and being seen with those, and, well, at one time I really didn't want to accept that either.' Pauline paused and thought about it. Yes, she'd sort of forgotten that, although she hadn't really. But she had come to terms with using sticks and crutches to balance. So it must be a similar kind of process, she thought.

'So you had similar kinds of feeling about using sticks . . .'

'Sort of around being seen by people, but there's, I don't know, something about being seated. That'll feel weird, I know it will. Daft, because here I am sitting down, but that's different, so different.'

'Yeah, you know what it's like sitting here, but out there, in a wheelchair, brings up all kinds of feelings and thoughts.'

Pauline was aware that her anxiety was increasing again. Dammit, she thought, I don't need that. But it is what I'm feeling about all this. 'Leaves me anxious again thinking about it.' Pauline could feel emotions welling up inside her. 'I've always tried to avoid this, keep this moment in the distance. Now it's so close, so horribly, horribly close.' At this, she broke down in tears.

Jim sat and responded quietly, 'Yeah, horribly close . . . horribly close.' He sat looking at Pauline who was sitting with her face in her hands.

'Oh dear.' She blew out a deep breath as she drew her hands away and reached for a tissue. 'I feel suddenly quite wretched again. Am I going through some feelings. I was feeling strong and determined just now and, well, look at me now.'

'Switches fast from strong to wretched and emotional.'

'Can't believe it and yet, well . . .' She shook her head. Yet she knew that this was how it had been and was probably going to continue for a while at least. And somehow she had to find a way through it, find a way to focus herself on what she needed to do. She sat quietly for a few moments, collecting her thoughts once again.

> People can switch mood very fast, particularly where they are trying to impose some new idea or action on themselves which other parts of their nature do not accept. Her determination, while clear and strong, is also quite fragile, like very thin glass perhaps. It doesn't take much to break it. As a person-centred counsellor Jim conveys his empathic understanding of what Pauline is saying and experiencing, not trying to rescue her. He knows that she must discover or maybe generate the inner resources that will enable her to sustain that determination. It has helped her through so much in her life. 'Individuals have within themselves vast resources for self-understanding and for altering their self-concepts, basic attitudes and self-directed behaviour; these resources can be tapped if a definable climate of facilitative psychological attitudes can be provided' (Rogers, 1980, p. 115). As a person-centred counsellor, this is fundamental and his responsibility is to offer that facilitative climate through his empathy, congruence and unconditional positive regard.

'Hard to believe, and yet all too familiar, yeah?'

Pauline nodded. 'Yeah, all too familiar.' She swallowed and took another deep breath. 'OK, I've got my focus back again. I need to …' she glanced at the clock, not much of the session left, 'I need to get myself together. I need to handle my anxiety better, and I have to not let myself get so down. Easy to say though.'

'Yeah, so, try and handle the anxiety better and not get so down. As you say, easy to say …'

'But I have to do it. And I know these are all parts of me, all these feelings, and yes, I feel anxious and I feel low, but I can feel strong and excited that maybe there will be positives in all of this. But I feel that I'm either really positive and enthusiastic, or really down and anxious, and never much in between. Real all or nothing, and I hate it. I hate the contrast as I drop down, as I feel the anxiety coming up. Hate it.' Her voice became quieter. 'I hate it.'

'Yeah, you hate it, mood down, anxiety up, struggling to hold on to any stability.'

'Don't seem to be able to do that much these days. But I guess, well, it's to be expected, you know?'

'It's a huge decision, and it's bringing so much of you, of your thoughts and feelings to the surface.'

'Yes, it really is.' Pauline was feeling suddenly very quiet. 'And it has to be, and I have to find a way through it, and it really helps having you here to talk to and to listen to me. I really mean that. I know I'm all over the place but I don't know how I'd have faced this otherwise. I really don't.'

'Thanks, Pauline, I appreciate that. And I'm kind of feeling that you'd find a way, but I'm glad to feel that I've helped, even though at times I realise how distressing it is, and how lost you feel in all of this.'

'Yes, but it's my distress. You help me become aware of it, help me get it out. That's what I need.' Pauline paused. 'God, I'm feeling tired again. It takes so much out of me. I'll be glad when I've got the wheelchair and can then get on with getting used to it, you know? I'm sure thinking about it, dwelling on it, doesn't help, or at least, I just keep getting stirred up about it, or feeling stuck in discomfort, you know?'

Jim nodded. 'Yes, maybe you'll feel different when you've got it.' Jim noted that it was a case of 'when' being voiced.

'I'm feeling a bit calmer now, but maybe that's because I don't think I've any energy left to feel anxious!'

> Pauline has engaged with such a wide range of feelings and through this process she is now once again sounding quite affirming of her intention to get a wheelchair and use it. The part of her that accepts this seems to be increasingly finding its voice, and while she is tired again at the end of the session, it seems that voice is getting stronger. She is talking about *when* she has it and her determination to get on with it. Her mood has switched around during the session, perhaps indicative of the fact of there being increasing parity between the accepting and the anxious parts of herself.

Jim smiled and nodded, and the session drew to a close. Jim was feeling tired as well. Again, it had felt very intense, and while he sensed Pauline edging ever closer to making a clear decision, he also appreciated that all of her wasn't completely accepting of the decision, and it might take a while longer before she took action. Or she might just act on impulse in a positive moment. It wasn't for him to encourage her either way. She needed to process this at her own pace and make her own choices when it felt right for her. But he did feel good that she had expressed appreciation for his help. Though, as was often the case, he wasn't always too sure exactly what he was doing, other than listening and attending, and holding his feelings of caring about Pauline. But then, as he knew, it was how he was with his clients that was so important, not so much what he did.

Points for discussion

- Reflect on your own feelings, thoughts and reactions to the last counselling session.
- How person-centred is David's supervision style? What seem to be his strengths, and what may be his weaknesses?
- Are there instances in the counselling session where you would have definitely responded differently to Pauline?
- How would your responses have differed and why?
- How present do you feel Jim was in this last session, and to what effect?
- How would you account for the speed at which Pauline switches from one frame of mind and set of feelings to another?
- Write your own notes for the last counselling session.

CHAPTER 8

Counselling session 8: the wheelchair – 'friend' or 'enemy'?

Four weeks have passed. Throughout that time, Pauline has continued with the counselling except for one week when she and Diana had gone away for a few days. She had been glad of the break. It had also made her realise how it might have been helpful to have had a wheelchair with them, particularly as she had a difficult couple of days when they were away. It hadn't been as difficult as some of her worse days; on those days she wouldn't have wanted to have gone anywhere, in a wheelchair or not. But they had been stiff and painful days, days when every movement seemed such an effort to make, and she hadn't slept well, and it had really been an effort to get about. They had gone to some gardens that actually had good paths and Pauline had felt frustrated that she hadn't been able to get around as much as she would have liked. It had made her a little more determined to get a powered chair, and they had also begun to look seriously at the possibility of a converted car so they could take it with them.

Jim had arrived on time and had walked up the path, and was ringing the buzzer. He could see some movement through the frosted glass so he waited for Diana to open the door. He heard Pauline's voice, 'Give it a push, it's unlocked.' He did so. It hadn't been Diana that he'd seen. It was Pauline, sitting grinning in a rather shiny, new wheelchair, with a high back support and, well, everything but the go-fast stripe down the side!

'Hey, wow, that looks great, and you're looking really pleased with yourself. You've gone for it! Yeah. Looks great. How does it feel?' Jim realised that he had maybe let his reaction run away with him, but Pauline was grinning and did look pleased, and it did feel right to be positive about it.

'Got it at the weekend. And it feels good, really comfortable. Better than I expected. I'm not using it all the time, but wanted you to see me in it, get your reaction.'

'Well, I feel like I want to give you a hug.' Jim just wanted to reach out and, yeah, give her a big hug. He didn't know what that was about, it didn't matter, just wanted to share what he was feeling, which was good. He walked down the hall towards her.

'Think I want to get up for this. I'm not having that bad a day today.' She got out of the chair, and Jim hugged her, gently but firmly, concerned in case he caused Pauline pain.

Jim took a deep breath as he stepped back. 'So, now the adaptation begins, yeah?'

'Sure does. I'm pleased I've got it. Just being able to get around when I want to, it does feel good. But I'm still walking. I don't want to spend all my time in it, and I'm going to go back into my chair now. But I just wanted you to see it, well, see me in it.'

'Well, I think it looks great, and I really hope it works out well, and, yeah, I guess it's going to be a bit of a learning curve for a while.'

'It seems pretty easy to manoeuvre.'

'Yes, I was thinking more about you and your getting used to it.'

They had returned to the lounge and Pauline was getting out of the wheelchair and returning to her own chair. 'So, what do you think?'

Jim noted the question. He felt his responses had communicated that but clearly Pauline wanted more, maybe checking out his response. He knew how important it was for her to sense other people's reactions and no doubt her thoughts and feelings, her concept of herself as a person in a wheelchair, would develop in response to how people reacted. And he had noted that she seemed to be feeling good about it, and that was important. She couldn't rely on the reactions of others solely. She needed to create her own sense of self.

Pauline is testing out her new identity with people she trusts, using their responses to build herself up. Jim's reaction is genuine. It encourages Pauline to feel good about being in the wheelchair. He isn't trying to make her feel good, he is simply being open with her. Feeling good about being in the wheelchair is a new experience. It is fragile and could easily be undermined by reactions that leave her feeling diminished in some way, and which could make it difficult for her to use it where the reactions of others are more unpredictable.

'I'm genuinely pleased, and I hope that it helps to make life a little easier for you, Pauline, I really do. I know how much of a huge decision it has been. I mean, the anguish, the range of feelings, the arguments either way going through your head, and the need to confront some of the stuff that left you unsure about it. But you've made the decision and, yes, I really hope it opens life up a bit more for you.' Jim was aware that he was grinning and half the time looking at Pauline, and the other half looking at the wheelchair. Pauline sat back down.

'Thanks. I feel good. I'm not as anxious as I was about it, not now I've got it. I'm amazed that I seem to have adapted quite quickly, but then, I'm like that. Once I make a decision I can move on quite, well, abruptly, I guess. It's like a new reality. I'm like that with moving home. Once I've made the move, that's it, I rarely dwell on what I've left behind, much more focused on the new reality. And that,' she turned to look at the wheelchair, 'is part of my new reality.'

Jim felt the urge to ask if she'd bought any spotlights for it, but decided against it. It was tempting to be flippant, the conversation felt easy, but he chose to stay with what Pauline had just said. 'Start of a new phase of life ...' Jim followed Pauline down the hall to the front room.

'And I'm sure there will be positives and negatives, but, well, that's always the case with anything new. So, there you are. I've done it now.'

'Yes.' Jim was curious as to what had happened because when he had seen her last time, though she was saying she had decided, she was still having a lot of anxiety.

'I'm aware of being curious as to what finally tipped the balance.' They were in the front room and Jim sat down. Pauline got out of the wheelchair and back into her usual chair.

'Ad in the paper. It's not new, although it's almost new. It was bought for a man who sadly died not long after getting it, and his wife was selling it. She didn't want it in the home, it reminded her too much of the past, and, well, we got a good deal with it. She was happy, said she felt pleased it was going to get used by someone who really would appreciate it, and we were happy, though we had to have some help getting it delivered – the batteries make it heavy – so a friend loaded it into the back of his transit and brought it over. Yeah. So. There it is.'

'Yeah, there it is.' Jim sat for a few moments continuing to look at it, then he brought his attention back to Pauline, smiling as he looked across to her and as their eyes met. They held the eye contact and, like in that earlier session, it felt a very powerful moment. Something important was shared; it felt to Jim like a kind of knowing, a sense of being allowed into the inner world of another person and yet no words were being exchanged. It felt like together they had reached a goal. It needed acknowledgement before moving on. 'Feels like you, we, have reached a goal. I want to acknowledge that.'

Pauline nodded and looked away briefly towards the wheelchair, and then looked back towards Jim. 'So, I'm not sure what to talk about today.' She shrugged her shoulders.

'I know it isn't one, a toy I mean, but there is something about how you are that reminds me of a child with a new toy.' Jim could see some sort of childlike reaction in Pauline. He realised it might be his interpretation, but it did somehow feel very real to him.

Pauline grinned. 'I know, and it's surprised me too. I keep getting in it and trundling around the place. When I'm doing that, I somehow feel good about it. But I have also found myself looking at it and wondering, am I doing the right thing? I mean, it feels right, but there are still doubts around.'

'Mhmm. Feels right when you are in it and there are doubts when you are not.'

Pauline was looking over towards the wheelchair. It still didn't look like it fitted in the room, somehow, all metal and black, and, well, it just stood out so much. Seemed to dominate the room, and she recognised that it was probably going to come to dominate her life as well.

'I'm just aware that I'm still very split on it, part of me resenting having to have it, another part of me excited about being able to move around more freely. But we've talked about that and, well, I guess I was kind of hoping my doubts would disappear once I had it. But they're still around.'

Jim was so conscious that Pauline had had the wheelchair for just a few days, and yet it had been an issue she would have dwelt on at different times for years. He fully expected her to take time even though, as she had said a little while back, she felt she could move on quite effectively and not keep looking backwards. 'So you have that sense of being able to move on and focus on the new reality and yet there is something about this that makes it difficult. You resent it, you're excited, you wish your doubts would have gone away.'

> Jim is drawing together Pauline's earlier comment about being able to move on, and her current experience of not being fully convinced. He offers his understanding of what Pauline has communicated as being present within herself.

'It's not like buying a house, or changing a job. It's . . .' Pauline was searching within herself to connect with what she was experiencing. She found it hard, it was hazy, and yet she had a clear sense of difference. 'I mean, when you move home, well, that's it, you're somewhere else and that is your reality and you start to adjust and adapt. I don't tend to look back in that situation. But this is different. And yet, it's not that I'm looking back.' She paused and grimaced. 'I don't know, it feels so difficult.'

Jim responded, 'It makes you grimace, something about this is very difficult.'

Pauline sat in silence thinking about it, but not really feeling she had any answer. It was somehow unsettling, though, not to be able to make sense of what she was experiencing. It just didn't seem clean, clear.

Jim sat with the silence, aware that he was experiencing discomfort himself. Maybe that wasn't quite the right word. But he did feel kind of sorry. At one level he knew that Pauline would need time to adjust, and yet he was sorry that she hadn't adjusted. He thought that odd as it was quite unrealistic, but he couldn't deny his own experience to himself. He sensed it to be his 'stuff' and put it to one side, making a mental note to reflect on it later. He brought his attention back to Pauline.

> Jim has chosen not to voice his experience of feeling sorry. His sense is that it is coming from his own 'stuff', that it is not emerging as a realistic response to what Pauline is saying. It's a professional decision on his part but it will need reflecting on.

'I'd like to feel that I can just see that,' she turned her face to the wheelchair, and back, 'as being reality. And at one level I know that it is, but something in me is still fighting it. It's like, I felt genuinely good greeting you in it. I really did. But once I was out of it sitting here, that sort of began to fade and now it's like it's ..., well, shit, this is stronger than I thought, but the word that comes to mind is "enemy".' Pauline could feel a sense of shock; it really was as strong as that and a huge contrast to how she had felt in the wheelchair when Jim had come in.

'So, what you're saying is that when you sit here looking at the wheelchair it seems like it is the enemy, but when you were sitting in it earlier when I arrived, you experienced it very differently.'

'Yes.' Pauline paused. A word had come straight into her mind. The polar opposite of enemy. 'It was my friend.' She lapsed into silence.

Jim felt the atmosphere change, although he couldn't describe the change in words other than there seemed to suddenly be a tension in the air. He concentrated his own focus, sensing that maybe something really important was happening for Pauline. He responded in a quiet voice, not wanting to disturb her silence and yet wanting to communicate that he had heard her, and so she could hear once again what she had said. 'Your friend.'

Pauline's thoughts had moved to medication. How many times over the years had she had that battle with herself? For years she had resented the tablets, the painkillers, the different medications trying to slow up the progress of the disease. How much she had fought against having to have them, not wanting to accept them, not wanting to feel that she needed pills to get about. It had been a hard lesson, and it had taken years before she had begun to come round to realising she had to work with the medication and not fight it, to begin to treat it more as a friend, there to help her, rather than as something external that she needed to cope with. She'd hated the idea of accepting the medication, even though the consultant, her doctor, friends and, well, everyone had been encouraging her to be grateful. But she hadn't been. Bloody pills. She hated the thought of being reliant on them. She hated feeling she was losing her independence. And she hated the idea of giving in to them or to anything. And now she had given in, and there it was, sitting there. And she knew she saw it as an enemy, but she also knew she had to see it as a friend. She had to.

Jim sensed that there was a lot going on for Pauline. She seemed very concentrated and lost in her thoughts. He wasn't going to disturb her now. He would sit and wait, allow her to be with whatever process was present for her.

The person-centred counsellor is working with the client's process. Thinking in these terms is helpful. The client has an inner world within which they are moving around. Arguably, successful therapy enables the client to move round more easily and openly. Jim respects the therapeutic importance of the client's process, of what is, if you like, 'going on for them'. Clearly it is important enough for Pauline to hold her attention. She is telling him, through her silence, that she needs to be with what is present for her.

'I've been here before, Jim.'

Jim wasn't sure exactly what she meant. His initial thought emerged out of his personal belief in reincarnation, but that didn't exactly feel right.

'Been where before, Pauline?'

'This issue of "friend" and "enemy". I saw the medication like that, as the enemy, for so many years and now I have learned to accept it as a friend, as a helper.'

'Mhmm.' Jim saw no need to repeat back what Pauline had said, so he kept his response minimal but maintained his attention.

Pauline looked away from Jim and she could feel her eyes welling up with tears. 'All my life I've fought enemies. My brother who bullied me mercilessly and always seemed to get away with it, my parents who seemed to be forever arguing and never had much time for me, realising I was gay, and going through a long period of seeing men as the enemy, fighting the disease, fighting the medication, fighting injustices towards disabled people, and now I have to make an enemy of that as well. And I know it isn't, not really, but I can feel myself wanting to fight it, fight back, and I can't. I have to accept it. But I hate feeling that I'm losing out to an enemy, hate it.' She sniffed and hunted around for a tissue. The tears were trickling down both her cheeks. She blew her nose. 'It's happening again. Why can't I just stop fighting, why do I always have to see things, people, as enemies?'

'Seems like it goes back a long way, but it leaves you with this unanswered "why?".'

'I don't want to make an enemy of the wheelchair, but I can feel in myself that something in me wants to. But it's not an enemy, it really is a friend.' She closed her eyes. It felt like years of struggle were rising up inside her. She realised, however, that this was somehow different. Back to different again, she thought. 'This, though, is somehow distinctly personal. It's not me and someone else, it's about me and my sense of who I am.'

'Who you are?'

'It's the final label that says "you are disabled". You don't have one of those,' Pauline gesticulated towards the wheelchair, 'unless you are. I mean, I am registered disabled, but that's different. That wheelchair is a symbol, a very visible symbol, that says something about me, and I have no control over how people will react.'

'I'm struck by the sense of it being personal and of how it relates to who you are.'

Jim speaks from himself, with his own emphasis and is clearly directing Pauline towards a part of what she has said – it may be helpful but it isn't empathic.

'Yes, and this may sound odd, but it feels right, it's more akin to my owning my gayness than accepting medication. Does that make sense?'

It did to Jim. 'Yes, because it is about identity, about, as you say, who you are.'

Pauline was nodding. 'Yes, who I am. OK, so my body doesn't work too good, makes it hard for me to get about, but me, the person who I am, that's not disabled.' Pauline could feel her voice getting stronger. 'And it makes me angry how people seem to want to label others in a way that can seem like it refers to the whole person, but actually it is just part of them.'

'Yes, you have a disability, your identity is greater than being "disabled", is that what you mean?' Jim had a sense of what she meant from his own background working with substance users, and how labels like 'addict' and 'alcoholic' could be so powerful and dismissive of people although they only referred to one particular behaviour, however dominant that might be.

'Yes. And I know I sometimes talk of myself as a cripple, but that's when I'm feeling really pissed off, you know. In reality, I know I'm more than skin and bones. OK, my body contributes to my sense of self, of course it does, but I want to be more than defined by my body's illness.'

'Bloody tough feeling your identity is defined solely by illness, and you don't want that.'

'No, but that's what that wheelchair can do. People will see me and that will be their first thought and, you know, part of me wants to say, "Hey, so I'm in this wheelchair, but that's the only difference we have! I'm just like you. Get to know *me*."'

'Yeah, get to know *me*!' Jim emphasised the 'me' in his response as Pauline had done.

Pauline took a deep breath and gritted her teeth as she let the air back out. 'But that wheelchair is only as much of an enemy as I let it be. But it's the reactions of other people I can't control, and that's important and there's part of me that thinks "fuck them, if they can't or won't see me as a person like them who just happens to have a physically disabling disease".'

'Fuck them if they don't want to see the person, *Pauline*, that is more than the disease and the disability.'

'And I don't really want to feel like that, but I have to, don't I? I mean, I've got to get on with my life, you know? I mean, I remember when I first started to go out with girlfriends, it took a while to be visible about it. Tending to go to gay bars and stuff, you know. But now, we're so much more open about it. I've got to think that way about this. At least I won't be judged like you are when you're gay; you can see it in people's faces. They don't think there is something wrong, crazy, weird because you're in a wheelchair. Though they may look away. Shit, I've done it myself in the past, felt awkward, you know? But I want them to see me. Me! Pauline.' She paused and her expression changed. 'Gay and in a wheelchair; all I need now is to become an alcoholic and that's it, full complement of societal stigma!' Pauline raised a slight smile.

Jim added, 'And have a mental illness . . .'

'Oh yes, forgot that, and that's another huge area that society, people, need to be educated about. How did we get on to this? Oh yes, it was me. Well, it would be, wouldn't it, we're here to talk about me!'

'That's true. So where does all this leave you, this sense of having two societal stigmas to address?'

Jim was aware that his comment about mental illness had distracted Pauline, sidetracked her, and he wanted to bring it back to her focus. He knew why he had said it; he had had a period working at a community mental health service and had learned, via the clients, how stigmatised they often felt. It was his frame of reference; he didn't need to have said it. He recognised his need to be more disciplined, particularly where the therapeutic exchanges get more conversational. He knew he found it too easy to kind of slip out of role.

'I've got to get on with it, but I think I'm going to see, through the gay network, how many people are in my position. Maybe there's a network out there. It isn't something I've thought about, but that wheelchair really does affirm an identity for me and I kind of want to meet others in the same place. I think that would be really good for me.'

'Yeah, get some support. And yes, as you say, a real sense that you have to get on with it.'

'Maybe it would seem more friendly if I painted it pink!'

Jim laughed. 'Maybe it would, maybe it would!'

The session drew to a close with Pauline saying she'd let Jim make his own way out. He walked down the hall and out into the fresh air. He felt he had a lot to think about. And he felt there was probably a long way to go for Pauline to unravel some of the powerful conditioning factors that had contributed to her structure of self.

It was later that Jim reflected again on that sense of feeling sorry when Pauline was talking about how difficult it felt coming to terms with having the chair. It began to dawn on him that maybe he had been placing too much of his own hope in her having a positive response to the wheelchair. He reflected on it, on and off, for much of the rest of the day and it was during the evening that he began to recognise how he had probably had more of an agenda than he felt he had, that he did carry a strong sense that she would be better off with a wheelchair to get out and about a bit more. He began to see how that was linked to his own nature – liking to be outside, going places, seeing things, not being stuck indoors. He realised that he hadn't picked that up about himself, although he knew it. But somehow he had maybe unwittingly sort of leaned more towards having the chair than not having the chair, and he was then unsure how that might have affected his empathy, his responding to Pauline, and what aspects of his own experiencing he had chosen to voice, and what not to make visible.

The more he thought about it, the more he was able to recognise that he was carrying a hope that Pauline would have the wheelchair and that it would prove helpful to her, to get her out of her home a little more. He knew that he had been feeling that way, he'd mentioned it in a supervision session, but he hadn't somehow really connected with it. He didn't think it had been strong enough to encourage Pauline, but there was the fact that she had made the effort to show him the wheelchair when he arrived, and with her sitting in it. Was that her need, or had she been meeting a need of his that she might have sensed in the session? He realised he needed to explore this in supervision.

Jim knew that as a person-centred practitioner he needed to be clear as to what was present within him. He sensed that he had a blind spot and it needed to be made more visible to him. Yeah, he thought to himself, I can only be congruent if I am truly and accurately in touch with my own process, with the flow of experiencing within me. I didn't notice this, and therefore I couldn't make a conscious choice whether or not to make it visible to the client. It would therefore be more likely to come out in other ways, perhaps through tone of voice, or selective empathy.

At the same time, and he was aware that he could be making excuses, he also felt that part of this reaction was maybe more a genuinely human response than an issue-driven reaction. He did want to see Pauline enhance her quality of life, as he hoped that everyone he worked with could achieve that. Hell, he wanted that for himself. And he also knew that not everyone did want this; many people wanted to stay as they were, fearing change. And as a person-centred counsellor he needed to be accepting of that. He realised however that perhaps the truth was that part of him accepted it, but another part wanted people to grow and develop to fuller capacity as human beings.

Jim acknowledged to himself how he often thought of the clients having different 'parts' to themselves, but he needed to maybe be more aware of himself in similar terms, and how different parts of the client related to different parts of himself. The image came to mind of a dance hall. It's like some people you dance with, some you don't, some you connect with, some you feel no attraction for or even feel pushed away by, or we push ourselves away. Every time we engage with a client, all the 'parts', the 'configurations within self' that make up how we experience ourselves to be, are active to a lesser or greater extent in their own ways. He knew his responsibility was to try to be as openly aware of all that was present within him, and know whether what he was experiencing was connected to his own values, experiences, hopes and fears, or whether it was more of a genuinely empathic response within himself to what the client was saying or experiencing. How he was in himself, which 'parts' of himself were most present at any time, would impact on the quality and nature of his empathy, and on the degree of therapeutic value his relationship would have with his client.

Points for discussion

- How might you have reacted had you been Pauline's counsellor, finding her in her wheelchair? Would your reaction have differed from Jim's and, if so, why?
- What are your thoughts and feelings about the impact of labels on people. How does labelling affect the development of an individual's self-concept?

- How did Jim convey unconditional positive regard and warm acceptance of Pauline during this session?
- At times the dialogue becomes conversational. What role does 'conversational counselling' have in therapy?
- Think about how Jim might present issues from this session in supervision.
- Looking back over all of the sessions, what key moments stand out for you as being highly significant in Pauline's process?
- Write your own notes for this session.

Pauline reflects on her experience of counselling

'I'm finding the counselling so helpful. It's just so good having someone listening and taking me seriously, and not being phased by my feelings and my struggles. Jim offers a calm presence, and I feel I can rely on that. It kind of gives me courage to explore, to be a little more open to myself. It's not easy, though, and there are times when it has left me so tired that I have wondered why I put myself through it. But I know that deep down it is right and timely.

'It has helped me make a big decision, to get the wheelchair. Yet it has also caused me to be aware of aspects of myself that, well, I guess I was aware of them, but they're sharper now. My need to struggle, to fight for causes, I can see goes a long way back, and has affected so much of my life, and I need time to explore this more. The seeing the wheelchair as an enemy, I need to address that as well. As I think I said in the session, I thought I'd dealt with that in relation to the medication, but it's still there, just finds something else to hook on to.

'It really has felt intense over the weeks so far, and I'm amazed how much I have explored, and how much feeling has been present in the sessions. But I put that down to Jim. He seems to give off some kind of signal to me that says it's OK to feel, to be distressed, to be how I need to be.

'I feel excited now about the sessions; I really look forward to them. I'm learning so much, and yet I'm not really being taught anything. It's a different kind of learning, my own learning about me, about who I am.

'The identity issue is another area that clearly needs a bit of unravelling. I would like to spend time in therapy addressing this. The more I try to affirm who I am by stripping away labels and roles, what am I left with? Who am I? What am I? I'm not just disabled, I'm not just gay, I'm not just a woman, I'm all of these things, and yet so much more as well. I want to really get to know myself. It feels energising even though it is tiring as well. And that's so contradictory, but then, I think I've learned that life does seem full of contradictions.

'So, I wonder, what next? I don't know. I want to carry on with the counselling for a few more months at least. I'm sure it is going to help me define who I am as a "wheelchair operative", who is the person at the controls.

'As I think back over the sessions, those moments of eye contact make an impression, and the silences, just being allowed to feel my own feelings and think my own thoughts, that felt strangely important. Weird, isn't it, something that's often called a "talking therapy" and yet those moments when nothing is said, not verbally anyway, seem to stand out. And that sense of my whole body wanting to cry, that was – oooh, I get goosebumps thinking about that now and I know the emotions are close. I need to appreciate how much my body has been through, adjust my attitude, be grateful, in a way, and sort of acknowledge that we're facing this together. Sound strange? Maybe it does. But that's how I'm feeling at the moment.

'Anyway, I'm glad I am having this experience. I feel sure I would not have made the decision to buy the wheelchair if it hadn't been for the counselling. It has definitely freed me up to think differently, to be a little more open and accepting, although that part of me that gets anxious about the effect of not walking so much is still around. I guess it will be for some time, maybe always, and I have to accept that as part of who I am too.

'So much to learn. So much to come to terms with. And I thought my issue was simply whether or not I should buy a wheelchair! Well, I've resolved that one, answered that question, but now, so many more questions of myself to explore.'

Jim assesses his experience of being Pauline's counsellor

'I've really felt privileged to work with Pauline, to be invited into her home and into her inner world of pain and suffering, of struggle, of sadness and emotion. So many themes have emerged over the sessions, so many areas for Pauline to connect with and explore. I have felt affected by her powerlessness, by her pain, and also by her determination and her will to keep on keeping on in spite of everything.

'I don't know what will lie ahead in the sessions to come. Issues have come up that may be addressed, but that is up to Pauline. I trust her process, that there exists a kind of inner wisdom that ensures that, if the therapeutic climate is provided, elements within the person that need to be addressed will come to the surface. The identity issue seems important, and her sensed need to build a more accepting relationship towards the wheelchair.

'What a huge step it has been for her to buy it, and the look on her face when I came through the door in that last session. I wish I'd had a camera. She looked so pleased, and I felt so pleased as well. Maybe I should have had a picture of my expression! I wonder what effect my reaction had on her. I may have been the first person to see her in it, other than Diana, who already knew her. Those first reactions can be oh so important. But I was pleased that my reaction was wholly genuine. I did feel good, and it was lovely seeing Pauline smiling. Makes me smile thinking about it.

'And I don't want to lose sight of the pain and the struggle as well, and the mixed-up feelings about it. I realise I may have unwittingly been sending signals encouraging her to go for the wheelchair, but I do feel she has done the right thing. I do know of people in similar circumstances who delay too long and their quality of life diminishes as they find it increasingly difficult to get out and about. And yet I understand, as well, the reasons people have for hanging on as long as they can to try and avoid having to accept being in a wheelchair. I guess everyone must make up their own mind and hopefully they make the decision that is right for them. Maybe if more people had counselling at this stage – not taking a problem-solving line but offering the client a therapeutic relationship and time to make sense of the different thoughts, feelings and motivations at work within them – maybe it would enable people to make the healthy choice that is right for them. People can feel overwhelmed by advice, sometimes contradictory, but often it is given out of another's agenda, or to make them feel better.

'The truth is, the decision to accept the need for a wheelchair is a difficult one for most people. Progressive disability does not necessarily lead to this, but for a great many people it does. And it's not like an accident where they may suddenly *have* to use a wheelchair; rather the person is faced with the prospect of having to make their own decision, resolve their own "if and when" and the internal reactions that can encourage the person to push it away.

'Anyway, I'm feeling good about the relationship I have with Pauline. I respect and admire her. She's finding her way through a challenging period in her life and I am glad that I can offer something that is helpful to her.'

Author's epilogue

This has probably been the most difficult book to write for me so far, given that the subject matter is close to my own experience, and has left me with lots to think about and process. As I mentioned at the start, my experience was in a family affected by one person's progressive arthritis disability, not MS. In writing this book I have deepened my understanding of the enormity of the impact that progressive disability has not only on the client, but on those closest to them, and also on the counsellor. My first counselling client suffered from arthritis and I saw her at home. I realise that today arthritis is less likely to progress to the point that a wheelchair is inevitable, but for sufferers from MS, where it continues to progress, then the likelihood is far higher.

Both of the fictitious clients in this book, Gerry and Pauline, touched into my own learned reactions. Both became very real to me as I wrote my way into their inner worlds. I am left with a sense of hope that the reader will find, through their therapeutic journeys, a fuller appreciation of the experience of facing progressive disability and that their own counselling practice will be informed by this. As a person-centred counsellor, that means being made more fully aware of myself in relation to the issue. It means having a fuller experience of what becomes present for me and understanding where it originates and what meaning it conveys.

Working with a person who is in pain and/or has a physical disability requires an openness to the fact that our client will have had experiences outside of anything that we may have encountered. To be, in effect, trapped in a body that is deteriorating and in pain, day after day, having to often struggle and battle for benefits, recognition, ability to access what everyone else would consider to be their right, takes its toll. The outrage that may be present can be enormous. The person, the human being, screaming for recognition in the face of another thoughtless 'does s/he take sugar?' demands to be treated with dignity and respect. People are people, whatever the shape, size, colour and functioning of their bodies. Sadly, in our world, it is not only those suffering from progressive disability who have to constantly battle to be heard.

I am sorry to end this book. I now wish I could continue Pauline's story, taking her through the challenges that she may now face in therapy as it reflects the challenges in her own inner and outer lives. It may sound strange, but I want to know what happens! Will she really adapt and find it within herself to accept her wheelchair as a friend? Will she get an adapted car so she can take the chair with her, and so extend herself on days out, or on holidays? Will her doubts strike back, leaving her rejecting of the wheelchair? What will her future be like? How will her condition progress? I hope she has a good life.

And having written the above, my thoughts go back to Gerry. What will his future be like? Will he, some day, be faced with his own version of Pauline's dilemma? How will his family cope with his progressive disability? How will he manage to keep going? Will he allow his family to be close to him in his struggle, or will he close them out? Different stages of life, different stages of their progressive disabilities and yet the thread of connection runs between them, the sense of *solidarity* that emerges where there is a common struggle. Having stood in Gdansk at the shipyard where Lech Walesa began the political solidarity movement in Poland, and having been touched by the atmosphere of the place, the word and concept of solidarity has had special meaning for me. I digress.

I hope the characters in this book have touched you. I hope that it has left you with a sense of how it can be when working with clients with these challenges. I hope it has left you with an appreciation of the role of supervision in ensuring that the counsellor remains healthy and that the relationship with the client is therapeutic. And what of the counsellors, Maureen and Jim? How different might they be as a result of their experience of working with their two respective clients? What image do you have of them? What of their characteristics do you sense as being present in you, and what is very different? How did their style of counselling leave you feeling? Were they helpful, or could they have been more attuned to their clients?

Imagine that you are the counsellor to both Gerry and Pauline. You see them both on the same day. What impact would your work with each have on your work with the other?

Progressive disability is a part of the human experience. Pain is a very personal, private and isolating reality. Having a companion, someone who gives you attention and who listens carefully, who can genuinely offer warmth and unconditional positive regard, and who has the capacity to be transparently present, offers therapeutic space. But it is more than space: in truth what most people want of a companion is time – time to feel heard, time to feel understood, time to share their highs and lows, time to feel acknowledged as the unique and valuable person that they are.

References

Bozarth J (1998) *Person-Centred Therapy: a revolutionary paradigm*. PCCS Books, Ross-on-Wye.

Bozarth J and Wilkins P (eds) (2001) *Rogers' Therapeutic Conditions: evolution, theory and practice*. Volume 3: *UPR, Unconditional Positive Regard*. PCCS Books, Ross-on-Wye.

Bryant-Jefferies R (2001) *Counselling the Person Beyond the Alcohol Problem*. Jessica Kingsley Publishers, London.

Gaylin N (2001) *Family, Self and Psychotherapy: a person-centred perspective*. PCCS Books, Ross-on-Wye.

Haugh S and Merry T (eds) (2001) *Rogers' Therapeutic Conditions: evolution, theory and practice*. Volume 2: *Empathy*. PCCS Books, Ross-on-Wye.

Kirschenbaum H and Henderson VL (eds) (1990) *The Carl Rogers Reader*. Constable, London.

Mearns D (1999) Person centred therapy with configurations of self. *Counselling*. **10**: 125–30.

Mearns D and Thorne B (1988) *Person-Centred Counselling in Action*. Sage, London.

Mearns D and Thorne B (1999) *Person-Centred Counselling in Action* (2e). Sage, London.

Mearns D and Thorne B (2000) *Person Centred Therapy Today: new frontiers in theory and practice*. Sage, London.

Merry T (2002) *Learning and Being in Person Centred Counselling*. PCCS Books, Ross-on-Wye.

Prochaska JO and DiClemente CC (1982) Transtheoretical therapy: towards a more integrative model of change. *Psychotherapy: Theory, Research and Practice*. **19**: 276–88.

Rogers CR (1957) The necessary and sufficient conditions of therapeutic personality change. *Journal of Consulting Psychology*. **21**: 95–103.

Rogers CR (1959) A theory of therapy, personality and interpersonal relationships as developed in the client-centred framework. In: S Koch (ed.) *Psychology: a study of a science*. Volume 3: *Formulations of the person and the social context*. McGraw-Hill, New York, pp. 219–35.

Rogers CR (1980) *A Way of Being*. Houghton Mifflin, Boston, MA.

Rogers CR (1986) A client-centered/person-centered approach to therapy. In: I Kutash and A Wolfe (eds) *Psychotherapists' Casebook*. Jossey-Bass, San Francisco, pp. 197–208.

Segal J (2002) Counselling people with multiple sclerosis. In: K Etherington (ed.) *Rehabilitation Counselling in Physical and Mental Health*. Jessica Kingsley Publishers, London.

Thorne B (1992) *Carl Rogers*. Sage, London.

Warner M (2002) Psychological contact, meaningful process and human nature. In: G Wyatt and P Sanders (eds) *Rogers' Therapeutic Conditions: evolution, theory and practice.* Volume 4: *Contact and Perception.* PCCS Books, Ross-on-Wye, pp. 76–96.

Wilhelm R (1968) *I Ching or Book of Changes.* Routledge and Kegan Paul, London, quoted in F Capra (1983) *The Turning Point.* Fontana Paperbacks, London.

Wilkins P (2003) *Person Centred Therapy in Focus.* Sage, London.

Wyatt G (ed.) (2001) *Rogers' Therapeutic Conditions: evolution, theory and practice.* Volume 1: *Congruence.* PCCS Books, Ross-on-Wye.

Wyatt G and Sanders P (eds) (2002) *Rogers' Therapeutic Conditions: evolution, theory and practice.* Volume 4: *Contact and Perception.* PCCS Books, Ross-on-Wye.

Useful contacts

Multiple Sclerosis Society UK
372 Edgware Road
London NW2 6ND
Tel: 020 8438 0700
Fax: 020 8438 0701
Email: webinfoenquiries@mssociety.org.uk
Website: www.mssociety.org.uk

Multiple Sclerosis Helpline Freephone
Tel: 0808 800 8000

The MS Society is the UK's largest charity dedicated to supporting everyone whose life is touched by MS. It provides respite care, a freephone MS helpline, grants for home adaptations and mobility aids, education and training, specialist MS nurses and a wide range of information booklets. Local branches cater for people of all ages and interests, and are run by people with direct experience of MS. The MS Society also funds vital research projects in the UK. Membership is open to people with MS, their families, carers, friends and supporters.

Multiple Sclerosis Society, Scotland
National Office
Ratho Park
88 Glasgow Road
Ratho Station
Newbridge EH28 8PP
Tel: 0131 335 4050
Fax: 0131 335 4051
Email: admin@mssocietyscotland.org.uk

Multiple Sclerosis Society, Northern Ireland
The Resource Centre
34 Annadale Avenue
Belfast BT7 3JJ
Tel: 028 9080 2802

Multiple Sclerosis Trust
Spirella Building
Letchworth
Herts SG6 4ET
Tel: 01462 476700
Fax: 01462 476710
Email: info@mstrust.org.uk
Website: www.mstrust.org.uk

The Trust offers information about all aspects of multiple sclerosis. It publishes quarterly newsletters: *Open Door* for people with MS, their families and friends; *Way Ahead* for health and social care professionals; *MS Information Update* bringing together abstracted details of recent research papers relevant to MS. Through its website it offers downloadable publications, professional education courses, expert chatrooms, discussion groups and links to other sources of information. The Multiple Sclerosis Trust also offers a Personalised Information Service to help people find answers to the questions that they have about any aspect of treatment, care or current research into MS.

Further reading

Etherington K (2002) *Rehabilitation Counselling in Physical and Mental Health*. Jessica Kingsley Publishers, London.

Rogers CR (1961) *On Becoming a Person*. Constable, London.

Index